LUPUS

What's It All About?

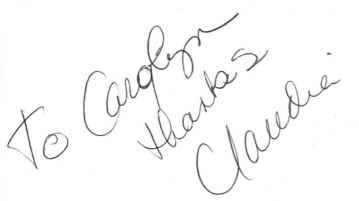

Books by Mary McClure Goulding:

Who's Been Living In Your Head?
A Time To Say Good-bye
Sweet love Remembered

Books by
Mary McClure Goulding and Robert L. Goulding:

Changing Lives through Redecision Therapy
The Power Is In the Patient
Not To Worry

LUPUS

What's It All About?

Claudia Pagano, R.N., B.S.N.
and Mary McClure Goulding, M.S.W.

Abiding Health Publications

Salinas, California

Library of Congress Catalog Card Number 97-77605.

Library of Congress Cataloging in Publication Data

Claudia Pagano, 1953 -
Mary McClure Goulding, 1925 -
LUPUS — WHAT'S IT ALL ABOUT? 1. Pagano, Claudia\
Goulding, Mary McClure 2. Lupus - United States -
Biographies 3. Disease: autoimmune 4. Women 5. Psy-
chology 6. Self-help 7. Health 8. Disability requirements.

Includes biographical material and an index.

Cover Design by Cynthia Heier
Interior Design by Printer Ready
Printed by Malloy Lithographing, Inc.

ISBN 0-9661036-3-7 51495

Abiding Health Publications
P.O. Box 3828
Salinas, CA 93912

Acknowledgements

I want to thank:

The Salinas-Monterey and the San Franciso subchapters of the Bay Area Lupus Foundation, with special appreciation for those who shared their life stories with us. You are all very dear to me.

David Wofsy, M.D.; Howard Press, M.D.; and Joan Barber, M.D. for their contributions to this book.

Jo Dewhirst, director of the Bay Area Lupus chapter of the Lupus Foundation of America, for her encouragement.

Joen Fagan, who helped us master the Internet, and then wrote about it.

Karen Edwards, Robert Free, and David Edwards for their moral support, helpful suggestions, and computer labor.

And especially my children, Brian and Ruth, with hopes that they will be a bit in awe of their mother now that she actually is an author.

Claudia Pagano

Contents

Warning

This book is designed to give information about lupus. Nothing in this book, neither the medical nor the non-medical information and procedures, are intended as a substitute for medical advice. Every lupus patient needs to be in the care of a physician. All matters regarding physical health should be supervised by a medical professional.

In medicine and in complementary treatment, new ideas emerge daily. There may be typographical mistakes as well as mistakes in content in this book. Although every effort has been made to make this book comprehensive, we ask readers to consider this text to be a general guide that is not a medical text.

The authors and Abiding Health Publications have neither liability nor responsibility for any loss or damage, caused or alleged to be caused, by information contained in this book.

The men and women with lupus tell their stories, but names are changed and disguises are used to allow them to be anonymous.

Introduction

This book is for the more than 600,000 women and 60,000 men in the United States who suffer from lupus. I write from firsthand knowledge. I am a nurse and also a lupus patient. As a nurse with lupus, I don't minimize suffering or pretend that only physicians know what is best for the individual.

Lupus is a strange and terrible disease. One day a person feels fine and the next day she can't get out of bed. She may have pain so excruciating that she spends the whole night in the bath tub, crying as she works to keep the water as hot as she can stand it. Another night, for no discernible reason, she may feel well enough to go dancing.

Lupus may attack a patient's kidneys, heart, or brain, or her only symptoms may be joint pain or that lupus rash on nose and cheeks. Lupus causes depression. So do some of the medications that treat lupus. Whatever the symptoms, lupus is a chronic and as yet incurable disease.

What is lupus? What are its manifestations and how is it diagnosed? Which physicians specialize in this disease? What medications do they use, and why? What about the alternative or complementary treatments? LUPUS — WHAT'S IT ALL ABOUT? answers these questions and many more.

Three physicians, lupus specialists, share their thoughts about lupus and lupus patients. A rheumatologist explains what a patient can do to help her physician provide her with the best treatment. An internist, who uses herbal medicine and acupuncture as well as traditional medicine, describes his holistic approach. A research physician shares the exciting research he is doing.

Psychological well-being is an essential part of lupus treatment. My co-author, Mary McClure Goulding, an internationally recognized teacher of psychotherapy, presents techniques for improving the quality of life by using breathing exercises, relaxation, imagery, and story-telling. She teaches assertiveness, and how to substitute self-caring for worry and unhappiness.

In the chapters, "Your Work Life" and "Your Home Life," everyday issues are presented and discussed, such as short cuts in housework and whether to keep your job or apply for disability benefits, plus a step by step guide to applying for these benefits. The mysteries of computer use are made easy, so that readers can join chat groups and get the newest information about lupus.

To me the most inspiring section in this book is "Women and Men with Lupus Tell Their Stories." Each lupus patient is unique, and responds uniquely to this disease.

One woman is now able to joke about a honeymoon that ended in her near-total paralysis, and tells of her long and successful struggle to regain mobility.

Four women, whose kidneys failed, describe their quite-different experiences with dialysis.

A woman who is legally blind, disabled, and almost seventy years old, survives on only $660 a month Supplemental Security Income, but nevertheless manages to go to college.

Some men and women are employed and others have been forced by their illness to quit their jobs. Some have children, some are childless, some have partners, and some live alone. Two women reveal how their marriages were strengthened as their husbands helped them cope with the trauma of lupus. Two women were deserted by husbands who wouldn't tolerate their disease, one while she was hospitalized in the intensive care unit. One woman ended a seven-year relationship with her lover, when she realized that she needed a more peaceful life than was possible with him.

A man, who couldn't even hold a glass or step over a tiny p on the sidewalk, put all his effort into an exercise pro- that made him strong enough to compete again in sail- es.

These women and men, Mexican-American, Black, Japanese-American, and White, belong to lupus support groups sponsored by the Lupus Foundation of America. They have become intimate friends, as they tell each other their joy and pain. I am one of them.

Although I was a registered nurse when I was diagnosed with lupus, I knew nothing about the disease. My physicians did the right tests and then prescribed the right medications, but when I mentioned that I needed fourteen hours of sleep every day, and that I often cried on the way home from a perfectly fine day at work, their faces went blank. Usually, they changed the subject.

I began reading everything that was written on lupus, and started a local support group for lupus patients. I wanted to learn what others did to cope with this disease. It's taken years, but I think I now understand what we lupus patients are going through physically and emotionally, and what we can do to optimize our health.

This book is my first, and the writing of it has been demanding and sometimes awesome. It's also been plain fun, especially when my family started sending ideas for book titles: Don't Be A Dufus, Read About Lupus. Thrown For A Lupus? The Straight Poopus On Lupus. The Lupusite's Guide To All Things Lupusitical. And, finally, Ask Not What Your Lupus Can Do For You, Ask What You Can Do For Your Lupus. It is a serious subject, and at times I can laugh about it.

My goal is to share what I have learned with lupus patients, families, friends, and health care providers, as well as with ill people who have not yet been diagnosed but think they might have lupus. All of these people are still trying, as I have tried, to find out:

LUPUS - - What's It All About?

1

What Is Lupus?

The official name of lupus is systemic lupus erythematosus, or SLE. It is a chronic, inflammatory disease that affects different parts of your body. For some unknown reason, your auto-immune system has gotten permanently out of whack. In addition to doing its usual job of attacking germs and other unwelcome invaders in your body, it has begun attacking your body's own tissues. It may be waging war against your skin, glands, bone marrow, blood, connective tissue, or such organs as your kidneys, heart, lungs, or brain.

The symptoms are confusing, contradictory, and ever-changing. You may feel pain in your hands and then in your gut, be very sick for days at a time and then suddenly become almost symptom-free, without having the slightest idea why your symptoms appear or disappear. That's the reason lupus is called "the disease with 1,000 faces." Each person's experience with lupus is unique, as you will see as you read what fourteen women and men say about their lupus in the following section.

What else about lupus?

It is a chronic disease for which there is no known cure. It is not contagious. You didn't get it from someone else, and you can't pass it on to your children, loved ones, or anyone. No one can catch lupus from you.

A few men get lupus, and very rarely lupus shows up in females before adolescence or after menopause; however, more than ninety percent of lupus patients, are women of childbearing age. No one knows why this is true, although researchers suspect that female hormones are in some way involved.

Since lupus is not contagious, why does one person get lupus and not another? Perhaps certain diseases, contracted earlier in a person's life, may leave her* susceptible to lupus. There may be genetic explanations. Lupus may be caused by a virus or a "cluster of viral influences." Environmental causes are a possibility. Researchers are looking carefully at patients' medical histories and also are seeking genetic, environmental, and viral causes. So far, unfortunately, the cause or causes remain undiscovered.

Hereditary factors are difficult to trace, because in the past lupus was rarely diagnosed. Although a very old disease, until quite recently lupus was known only to rheumatologists and the type of physician whose hobby was reading about esoteric illnesses.

Now, every physician in America, and many lay people, know of lupus. In the United States today it is estimated that more than 600,000 women and about 60,000 men have systemic lupus erythematosus. More than 15,000 new cases are diagnosed each year.

Before lupus was well-known, physicians and the general public used to say, "She's just the ailing type," or "She was born weak," or "It's all in her mind." Surely, these remarks did not do much to make the life of a lupus sufferer happier. Imagine what it is like to be unable to get out of bed, or to hurt in every joint, and be told you are just weak or neurotic. Even today women are called "hypochondriacs" when their diseases cannot be diagnosed. A number of these women suffer from lupus.

Lupus is difficult to diagnose because of its changing and contradictory symptoms. No one has all of them, but all lupus patients have some of them from time to time. Most people with lupus have experienced the big four: exhaustion; pain, usually in the joints; sun sensitivity; and that red rash that sup-

---

* In the past male pronouns were used to designate men and women. Because most lupus patients are women, in this book the female pronouns may refer to both male and female patients.

posedly reminded a French physician, almost 150 years ago, of "wolf bites on the face." Where in the world did he see people with wolf bites on the face, especially bites that didn't break the skin? Other medical historians believe that he named the disease lupus because the rash looks like the darker shadings on a wolf's face. Anyway, lupus is Latin for wolf.

That French physician wasn't the first to discover lupus. Good old Hippocrates described the rash in about 400 BC.

If you suspect that you may have lupus, read the list of symptoms to see if some of them apply to you.

Malar Rash. This red rash, for which lupus was named, appears over the bridge of the nose and across both cheeks. If you are the type of person who likes to imagine that rashes look like something other than just a rash, its form might remind you of a butterfly. It may be visible for only an hour or two, or for days or weeks. Usually, it comes and goes.

(Some people get a different rash, round and scaly spots that may show up on any part of the body exposed to the sun, though it, too, is most common on the face. If it isn't treated, it may leave white spots or scars. This is a different disease, called discoid lupus.)

Sun Sensitivity. You may notice your rash for the first time after you've been in the sun. You think you have a sunburn, except that it is different from sunburns you've had before. Instead of pealing or turning into a tan, it remains red and may have raised patches. Perhaps you were healthy until you got a mild sunburn, and then the burn turned into welts and your joints began to ache.

The sun is your enemy. Whether or not you have been a sun lover in the past, your days of seeking the perfect tan are over. Even short exposures to the sun may make your symptoms worse. And it's not just bright sun. Any exposure to the sun's UVA and UVB rays, such as those reflected off sidewalks, sand, or snow, are harmful to you. If you are one of the minority of lupus patients whose skin is not sensitive to the sun, you may believe that the sun is good for you, because its heat on your body makes your joints feel better. The truth is, no matter what is happening to your skin, the sun's rays are stimulating the production of auto-antibodies which activate your lupus. You cannot be outside even on cloudy days without a long-sleeved shirt, sun hat, and gloves, especially between 11 am and 3 pm, when the sun's rays are strongest. For some people, even prolonged exposure to halogen lights or copy machines may cause a lupus flare.

Pain. Lupus pain may be very mild or may be terrible. "I hurt all over," some say. One adolescent told her physician, "Even my hair hurts." The pain may be sharp, a steady ache, or a burning sensation, and it probably is located, like arthritis, in your joints, especially the joints of hands and fingers. Some people also have swelling and tenderness in their joints. Some have pain in their muscles rather than their joints. The pain may move around. One day it is in your ankle and the next day in the back of your neck, and another day it is everywhere. Or you may be lucky and not have much pain at all. Even if your pain is severe, it is not constant and your physician can prescribe medicine that will bring you relief, so don't despair!

Exhaustion. Exhaustion, like the pain and the rash, comes and goes, and almost always is worse during the early stages of your illness. What's the exhaustion like? In your pre-lupus days, you may have been the sort of person who raced home from work, grabbed a mountain bike and rode ten miles before supper. Or you may have ended the day tired, but able to go to the grocery store, fix supper for the children, and throw a load of laundry in the washer before you collapsed in front of the TV.

Lupus exhaustion is something new. As Tom (chapter 15,) said, "All of a sudden, I got so tired I'd even have to rest on my way back from taking out the garbage. How do you explain to anyone that you can't take out the garbage without resting?"

You may wake up in the morning too tired to get out of bed. Other days you go to work, but you have to lie down almost as soon as you arrive. On the way home from work, you pull over to the side of the road to nap, before you can continue your drive home. On bad days, grocery shopping and cooking are impossible, and doing anything with children beyond reading to them is from another lifetime. You may be too tired even to hold a book.

Again, everyone is different. Some people feel vaguely tired, but can carry on their usual activities. One of the strange aspects of this disease is that the exhaustion, for no known reason, comes and goes. You may not be able to get out of bed one day, and the next day you are again energetic.

Later, when you and your doctor have figured out what medications are best for you, and when you have learned some simple ways to reduce stress and care for your body, you'll get back your enthusiasm for living. You still will need lots of sleep. Most people with lupus sleep at least ten hours out of every twenty-four.

There are other symptoms besides the four most prevalent ones:

Depression. Depression is common in lupus patients. Anyone who suffers the pain and exhaustion of lupus might be expected to be depressed, but a lupus depression is more than simply a response to a chronic and very difficult physical illness. It seems to be organically based, meaning that your body produces your depression, just as it also produces rash, exhaustion, or pain. The classic symptom of this type of depression is an overwhelming feeling of despair. Patients may or may not verbalize this despair, but the words that go with such despair are, "There's no hope for me," "Nobody can help me," and "There is nothing worth living for."

In reality, there is help and hope for you, and you'll find much to live for. A lupus depression is curable, but in the midst of your depression, you may not believe this.

Easy Bruising. You don't know that you bumped your arm or leg, until you see your black and blue bruises. Sometimes lupus medication causes this condition, but it may also be a sign that your lupus is attacking the platelets, which allow your blood to clot.

Hair Loss. You notice that your comb or brush are full of hair, and you may find hair on your pillow. This is an occasional occurrence during lupus flares, and won't be continuous.

Fever. Some people run a consistent low-grade fever, perhaps 100 degrees. Others run high fevers that come and go for no apparent reason. Check your temperature when you think you are running a fever.

Chest Pain. You may feel a sharp pain in your chest that is not a heart attack. Usually, the cause is inflammation of the connective tissue between your ribs. However, the pain may be due to inflammation of the lining of your heart or your lungs. This needs immediate treatment. A physician can differentiate easily between heart, lung, and connective tissue inflammation.

Edema. If your kidneys are affected, one of the first signs is swelling (edema) of your legs, ankles, and feet. You may see in the mirror that there is also swelling around your eyes. Again, see a physician right away, preferably a nephrologist, a physician who specializes in kidney diseases. Early treatment can save your kidneys.

Cold hands and feet. As with other lupus symptoms, coldness in the extremities can be caused by a variety of physical problems, so it is not by itself a test for lupus. If your fingers turn white when cold, and bright red when warmed, you may have Raynaud's syndrome, or Raynaud's and lupus together.

Dry Eyes and Dry Mouth. This symptom occurs in about ten percent of lupus patients, and sometimes means that your lupus is involved in the glands that produce saliva and tears. You may have Sjogren's syndrome, a different, usually quite mild disease that often accompanies lupus. Or, as with other symptoms, your dry eyes and mouth may be caused by something that has nothing to do with lupus.

Confusion. Driving your car, you suddenly don't know where you are going, or how to navigate streets that in the past you knew well. Routine jobs you've done dozens of times become impossible to figure out. Usually your confusion is short-lived, but for some people it hangs around for a longer time. Some medications can clear up confusion, and others actually cause it. No wonder lupus patients need good doctors and lots of emotional support! If you have symptoms of confusion, you need someone to help think for you, so you don't make precipitous decisions, as Vera (Chapter 9) did, when suddenly she couldn't remember how to run the computer at work. She fled from her job out of fear and shame, instead of taking the sick leave she deserved. In a short time, her memory returned, but it was too late to get her job back.

Neurologists are finding other symptoms in addition to confusion, including inability to remember words, co-ordination difficulties, and headaches. These symptoms, now grouped together, are called neuropsychiatric lupus.

Pre-Menstrual Flares. Whatever your lupus symptoms, you will probably notice that premenstrual flares are common. Just before your period is due, your symptoms become worse. You'll learn to take special care of yourself, and not plan difficult or taxing activities at this time each month.

Those are the common symptoms of lupus. To know which symptoms apply to you, you need to be aware of your own body and what is going on with it. Perhaps in the past you were a person who took your body for granted. Most people do. From time to time they exercise, go on diets, or lie in the sun to get a good tan, but mostly they don't concern themselves with their bodies. If you have lupus, you must concern yourself with your body. Your life may depend on it.

No one has every symptom, and each of the symptoms, seen alone, can point to problems other than lupus. If you have three or four of these symptoms, or if any one of these symptoms is severe, you'll want a physician to order laboratory tests to help diagnose your illness.

A few people with lupus, especially those who are on steroids for treatment of other diseases, have such minor symptoms that they hardly even know they have the disease. Others feel very ill right from the beginning. In the past, the majority of lupus sufferers died within a few years, but today almost everyone with lupus can live out a full, active life. You can, too, especially if you and your physicians do a good job of taking care of you.

Probably you don't need urging to make an appointment with your physician. Even if in the past you've been the type to avoid doctors, this time you know from your level of pain, fatigue, and general distress that something is very wrong with you.

But when you get to the doctor's office, you may feel much better and your rash may have subsided. You may be a bit embarrassed that you are taking a physician's time with something that has already "gone away." On the other hand, you may be too exhausted and depressed to explain satisfactorily what you are experiencing. It may seem hard to speak convincingly about how much you hurt or how tired you are.

In order to give a complete report to your physician, re-read the list of symptoms, and write down all of them that you have experienced, plus any others that are not listed. That way, you'll be able to present a clear picture of what has been going wrong with your body.

Although no one can cure your lupus, much can be done to alleviate your symptoms and prevent permanent damage to your vital organs. Remember, more and more studies and experiments are being undertaken to find new ways to treat systemic lupus erythematosus. In the future, who knows what new treatments or even cures will be available? If you and your physicians do everything possible for your health today, you'll be ready as the newer and better treatment methods arrive.

In the following chapter you will learn more about how physicians diagnose and treat systemic lupus erythematosus. You'll learn which medical specialists you need, and how to find them. You'll learn about medications, as well as complementary or "new age" medicine. In addition, you'll discover many simple, enjoyable, and effective methods for helping yourself.

You'll also get to know some lovely, exciting women and men, who report on how they have managed to live with lupus. Each person describes her particular symptoms, and her own unique methods of coping with problems at home and at work. They are members of lupus support groups, which meet regularly to share information about lupus, and have fun together.

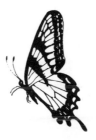

2

Finding A Doctor And Getting A Diagnosis

First of all, let's assume that you have some symptoms of lupus, and are looking for a good physician. Perhaps you have a primary care physician. You may want to see this person for your first appointment, or you may have no choice for the first appointment. If you are hurting badly and have frightening symptoms, you don't want to dally around, looking for a new physician. It is understandable that you need someone right now. With luck, you have a primary care physician whom you like and find easy to talk with.

If not, make an appointment with a rheumatologist, because these doctors specialize in diagnosing and treating lupus. Remind yourself that you can choose a new physician at any stage of your treatment. More about that later.

Now you need to prepare for your appointment. In the old days, that meant only that you should take a bath and wear clean, nice underwear so that the doctor would think well of you. That was what your grandmother was told, when she was a child. In her world, her family doctor knew her entire family well, and made treatment decisions that everyone obeyed. In today's world, the practice of medicine is more technical and scientific - - actually, it is far better medicine - - but physicians are busier, may not know your family or you, and they definitely need your help.

You can do your part by gathering the necessary medical information ahead of time. Before your appointment, write down your family medical history, your medical history, a list of past and present medicines that have been prescribed for you, your current symptoms, and your questions about your symptoms. Use four sheets of paper.

On the first sheet, write the significant diseases that members of your family had. If you don't know what is significant, put down all the diseases you remember. Include on the list the causes of death of your grandparents, parents, aunts and uncles, and brothers and sisters.

On the second sheet of paper, write your own medical history. Write the names of all illnesses and all surgeries you have had, with approximate dates, as well as the names and phone numbers of physicians you have seen recently. If you are allergic to any medicine, don't forget to list it, too! List each medicine you are currently taking, the dosage, and how long you have been taking it. Also list medicines that you have taken during the past year or two, and are no longer taking. If you are uncertain of the names of these medicines, put all your medicines in a bag and bring them with you.

On the third page, list the symptoms that you have experienced during the past month. Re-read the symptoms listed in the first chapter of this book, to help you remember, and be sure to write down any symptoms that are not on that list. Underline the symptoms that led you to make this appointment, the ones that are especially troublesome or painful.

The fourth sheet of paper, which you need for every visit no matter how often you see a physician, is your list of questions. Always, keep a written list of questions that you want to discuss with your physician. Otherwise, during a brief, hurried appointment, you may forget them.

Now that you have the information your physician will seek, plus your own questions, you need to put yourself in the right frame of mind. Some people are afraid of doctors because of past experiences, or because their parents were afraid. Some go into a doctor's office as if they are peasants being brought before the King or Queen. It is important that you maintain your self-esteem and dignity. Ignorance and poor self-esteem lead to poor treatment and, therefore, a worsening of your symptoms.

Tell yourself, as you walk into the office, "I am not a little child. I am a competent adult." You are not in a physician's office to please the physician, or to prove that you are sweet, lovable, respectful, or brave. Remind yourself that the physician is neither your parent nor your god. You don't have to prove that you are ill. You already know that fact. You are there for the physician to use her* expertise to diagnose your illness correctly and begin treatment. You are there to get relief from your symptoms.

You are keeping an appointment with a physician in order to receive expert help for your body. It is similar to seeking expert help for your home, if the roof leaks or there is a strange odor under the house. Whether you are hiring someone to repair your body or your home, you are in charge. You are talking to a doctor who is your employee, not your judge. And you will decide whether to continue to hire this person or seek another physician.

Someone in the physician's office will ask for your family history and your personal medical history, and, of course, what is troubling you that led you to make this appointment. You will take out your notes, and begin.

(If, after you have been seen by your doctor, she merely suggests "rest and aspirin," find another doctor immediately. Even today there are physicians who overlook the disease of lupus, or the seriousness of the disease. They still believe that their patients are depressed or hypochondriacal. These doctors should be avoided like the plague!)

Your physician will conduct a physical examination. In addition to the usual physical examination you've had lots of times, this physician will pay special attention to the areas of

---

* In the past almost all physicians were men. Male pronouns were used when referring non-specifically to men or women. Now many physicians are female, and in this book female pronouns will be used to designate male and female physicians.

your complaint. She will be checking for signs of lupus. She will look for oral ulcers, which have the appearance of cold sores and are caused by inflammation. To give an example of the contradictoriness of lupus symptoms: some patients have oral ulcers so small that physicians can't see them, but they hurt so much that patients know exactly where they are; other patients have large, painless ulcers they didn't know existed.

The doctor will palpate for tenderness around joints and areas of suspected inflammation. Your legs will be checked for signs of swelling. The doctor will examine your rashes, and order a biopsy if there are welts. Some lupus patients have serositis, which is an inflammation of the linings of heart, lungs, or intestines. The physician will listen through a stethoscope placed on your chest, for abnormal sounds such as those made by fluid, rubs (friction), or murmurs.

After the physical examination, your physician will order lab tests, and prescribe medication for relief of your symptoms. There is no reason for you to keep on hurting. You do not need the results of tests to be given medication for symptomatic relief.

Laboratory work is necessary for diagnosis; lupus is well known for mimicking other diseases, so you may seem to have lupus when in fact you have something else. You need tests that are specifically designed to find the lupus autoantibodies, as well as tests that will specifically rule out rheumatoid arthritis, AIDS, Lyme's disease, leukemia and lymphoma, neurologic disorders, tuberculosis, chronic fatigue syndrome, and other diseases.

You may be hospitalized for the laboratory work or you may be able to have the work done as an outpatient, depending on the severity of your symptoms.

Perhaps your doctor prefers not to order these tests but instead immediately refers you to a specialist: an internist, dermatologist, nephrologist, rheumatologist, neurologist, or cardiologist, depending on your symptoms. The specialist will order these tests.

A complete blood count is necessary. You've had this test before, because it is given as part of most annual physical exams. This time, the physician is on the alert for a low white blood cell count, low red blood cell count, or a lower than normal level of platelets. A low red count will show that you are anemic, and the cause might be lupus. About half of all lupus patients have a low white count and/or low platelets, which indicates a chronic, active disease.

Blood chemistry tests, which differ from the complete blood count, will be ordered to assess liver and kidney function, nutritional adequacy, and the presence or absence of infection.

ANA (antinuclear antibody test) is performed on serum from your blood. It is an important test for diagnosing lupus. The titer (strength) of the ANA gives an indication of the severity of the patient's disease, as it shows the presence of antinuclear antibodies in the bloodstream. Not all positive ANA tests indicate autoimmune disease; in fact, some perfectly healthy people have a positive ANA. If your ANA is positive and they suspect lupus, more specific autoantibody tests will be performed, such as Anti-Smith, anti-DS DNA to predict which organ systems may become endangered from your lupus.

A urinalysis will be ordered, to check for diabetes as well as to look for the presence of protein, or red or white blood cells in the urine, all of which are signs of impairment of the kidneys. To diagnose lupus nephritis (kidney disorder), the physician will do a urinalysis, including an analysis of a twenty-four hour urine collection, blood studies, and perhaps an Xray to determine the size and shape of your kidneys. Sometimes a biopsy is needed to assess the extent and severity of kidney disease.

You will be given a serologic test for syphilis. For some reason, a false positive result on this test is an almost sure sign of lupus. A false positive result means that the test says you have syphilis, but you don't have it. On the other hand, you can have a negative result and still have lupus.

Because lyme disease and systemic lupus erythematosus have very similar symptoms, it's a good idea to run the lyme titer test. Unfortunately, some lupus patients get a false positive result, so a follow-up blood test, called Western Bloc, will have to be ordered.

If the results of any of these tests indicate the possible presence of lupus, other tests may be ordered, such as complement level, sedimentation rates, and tests that have names like addresses on E-mail: IMM006.JPG, IMMOO7.JKPG, 1MMO10.JPG, etc.

In 1982 the American College of Rheumatology issued the criteria for establishing a diagnosis of Systemic Lupus Erythematosus. Officially, to be diagnosed with SLE a patient must have four of the following eleven criteria, though not necessarily at the same time:

1. Butterfly (Malar) rash
2. Discoid lesions, the reddish, raised patches that leave scars. If this is the only symptom, the diagnosis is discoid lupus rather than SLE.
3. Photosensitivity, specifically, a rash following exposure to sunlight.
4. Ulcerative sores in the mouth.
5. Arthritis with joint pain, tenderness, and swelling.
6. Evidence of either pleuritis or pericarditis: inflammation of the membranes lining the chest cavity or surrounding the heart.
7. Evidence of renal or kidney disorder.
8. Signs of a neurologic disorder: seizures, psychosis, or acute loss of memory, occurring without any other explanation such as drug toxicity or injury.
9. Hematologic abnormalities: specific deficits in various types of blood cells.

10. Immunologic disorders: false-positive reaction to the test for syphilis, positive LE cell test, presence of anti-DNA or anti-SM antibodies. Any one of these constitutes an immunologic disorder.

11. Abnormal level of antinuclear antibodies.

To prepare for your second medical visit, in which you will learn the results of your laboratory work, you should up-date your list of symptoms and include changes you've experienced in the symptoms, reactions to the medicines you were given, and all of your questions. You should be feeling much better, because at your first visit your doctor will have prescribed medication for the relief of your symptoms.

When you are faced with a potentially serious disease, or when you are feeling very ill, it's hard to concentrate on what a physician is saying. For that reason, it is a good idea to take a friend with you for this important second visit, so that both of you can understand what is being said. It is also a good idea to bring a tape recorder. The two, a friend and a tape recorder, can prove to be invaluable.

Your physician will want to know if your medication has been effective, and if you have had any side effects. She'll tell you the results of your laboratory tests. Perhaps she will order more tests.

Do not pretend to understand your doctor when she uses words that are unfamiliar to you. Ask her what these new words mean. Ask her to use words that you understand. Do not let yourself be intimidated by your own lack of knowledge or your fears of doctors or diseases. If you don't have a tape recorder, write down the laboratory results and the physician's explanation of them. Ask, "And how would I look this up at the library?" Explain that you want to read about your illness. Ask, "Does everyone call this medicine and this disease by these names, or are there other names that lay persons use?" It is important that your physician listen to you, believe you, and address each of your concerns.

If your doctor cannot establish a diagnosis of lupus according to the accepted eleven criteria, she may continue your medication and simply wait to see what develops. She may say you have "a connective tissue disorder," which is a very general term for what may or may not be lupus. That is, of course, frustrating for you, but often symptoms do not point clearly to a diagnosis. Although it is natural to want immediate answers, sometimes they aren't forthcoming, because the tests are not always definitive.

Physicians don't want to label your illness prematurely, treat you for an illness you don't have, or subject you to a false diagnosis that may remain attached to your medical record forever.

Whatever your diagnosis, you may choose to get a second opinion. If your physician is not a specialist in lupus, ask for a consultation with a specialist.

Your local lupus society has a list of physicians who specialize in the treatment of lupus. Get the list, and then ask health professionals in your area, such as nurses or medical social workers, "What doctor would you want for your loved ones, if one of them had the symptoms I have?"

You want a rheumatologist to go over the test results, because rheumatologists specialize in treating patients with lupus. Afterwards, you may continue with that specialist, or seek a different one. If you have severe kidney involvement, you will be referred to a nephrologist. In addition, you may need to see other physicians for specific problems. With neurological disorders you'll be referred to a psychiatrist or neurologist. If you have mouth or jaw pain, see a dentist with experience in treating lupus, because lupus patients' jaws sometimes develop changes that cause great pain until treated by a dentist who knows about this problem.

A few lupus patients develop *vasculitis*, an inflamation of blood vessels. This can occur in your eyes, kidneys, brain, abdomen, and almost anywhere in your body. If you have eye problems, vasculitis, or are taking the drug Plaquenil, you need to regularly consult an ophthalmologist who can visualize "cotton wool spots" on the back of your eyes which are caused by vasculitis.

You have a right to the best medical care you can find. Physicians have chosen their vocation because they want to help people live well. They want to save lives. Basically, they care deeply about their patients, and they have spent hard years learning to do their jobs to the best of their abilities. With a chronic disease, you want to have confidence in your physician, and know that the two of you can work well together. It's going to be a long, difficult road, which is infinitely easier when you travel it with someone you trust.

In the following fourteen chapters, women and men with lupus tell their own unique stories of their struggles with both the symptoms and the disease itself.

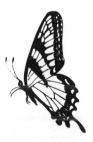

3

Pamela
I Hang My Dialysis Bag On The Rear View Mirror, And I'm Off

In spite of lupus, I'm doing fine. I have my ups and downs with it, and especially have flares in summer, even though I wear sun screen and big hats and everything, but lupus doesn't hold me back.

I don't have functioning kidneys any more, so I dialyze myself every night while I sleep. It's not a big deal. To use a home machine, you have to be self-motivated and be willing to understand how to keep yourself clean. The dialysis unit at the hospital tests my blood once a month to make sure the dialysis is working well, but if anything goes wrong, I know it before they do. All I have to do is put antibiotics into the dialysis bag, and that solves the problem. When I travel, I dialyze myself manually, of course. For instance, when I am driving, I just hang my dialysis bag over the rear-view mirror, and I'm off!

My husband Mitch and I go to San Francisco almost every other weekend to visit our friends and family, and last month we flew to Disneyland. On planes, I hold my bag over my head, and let it drip away merrily. So what if people wonder what I am doing? I am not embarrassed any more. I want to go places, and I refuse to stop having fun just because I have lupus. Do you understand? I'm still young and I'm not going to act like a sick old lady.

I even went white-water rafting this summer. I shouldn't be in the sun and I should never be in river water because of possible pollution. You see, I do peritoneal dialysis and that means I have a tube in my abdomen. I did bind myself well; I was good about that. As soon as I got out of the raft, I disinfected the tube and the skin around it, and I did not get infected! It was wonderful, but the dialysis unit thinks I am crazy to take risks, so I won't do it again.

I found out I had lupus when I was in college. At first I thought I overdid it in a volley ball game. My friends and I played a lot of volley ball in those days. I was nineteen and had just met Mitch at a dance. The evening of our second date, I was in the hospital. I didn't want to tell him I was sick, so I phoned and tried to make up excuses for not seeing him that night. He was upset, because he thought I didn't like him, or something. He kept asking, "Why aren't you coming with me tonight? Did I do something wrong?" Finally, I just blurted out, "If you must know, I can't go on a date with you because I am in the hospital." He came right over to the hospital to visit me there. That's how our romance started.

I was in the hospital because I had horribly high blood pressure from the lupus, and my kidneys weren't good. After that, I had to cut back on my college classes and it took me seven years to get my degree. I was on a very strict diet, and had to learn a lot about food. I figured I might as well get some advantage out of studying food, so I became a dietician. My kidneys were failing from day one, but with a strict diet, I managed to keep them functioning for more than ten years after I was diagnosed.

In the beginning, Mitch's family wasn't crazy about the idea of him marrying me. They wanted grandchildren and they thought he should have a wife who could work as hard as he did. You know how Chinese families are. I want children, too, but it's impossible, and fortunately Mitch is satisfied without children. Before we were married, his family got to like me in spite of my lupus.

I don't act sick when I am with our family or friends, so nobody remembers my lupus until I have to go to the hospital. You see, I've always been a happy person. Being sad doesn't make you well, so you might as well be happy. That's how I feel about it. Many people with lupus are depressed, but I'm not. Geez, there are lots more terrible diseases than lupus, diseases that kill you, for instance.

I refuse to let anything get me down and Mitch is even more of an optimist than I am. Sometimes at night I start to worry, and then he says, "Are you worrying about something you can fix tonight?" I say, "No," and he says, "Then go to sleep!"

I used to worry that I was a drag on him, but he says "Who else in the whole world would feed me as well as you do?" He's an easy-going guy who loves my cooking, and I am a very good cook.

When I tell him that I am a burden because I can only work part-time, he reminds me that he doesn't want me to work at all. It is important in Chinese families that the man be the one who makes most of the money. He has a good job, we have enough money, and we have lots of friends.

If I start wishing I could have children, he takes me to spend the weekend with my nieces and nephews, and they wear me out. Then I remember that I really couldn't handle both children and lupus. Our cat is our baby.

Nowadays, I don't have as much pain as lots of lupus patients have, but I still have to pace myself. If I walk too much, my ankle starts to hurt, and then I have to rest the next day. I can do anything and eat anything. It's a big improvement over the days when I was trying to save my kidneys.

I'm on the list for a kidney transplant. That scares me, but I want the transplant so that we can visit Hong Kong before the take-over by the mainland Chinese; and later I plan to go to Europe. Mitch and I can't carry all the dialysis stuff I'd need for a long trip. Travelling would be easy if I could avoid dialysis.

I have a very happy life.

Three months ago Pamela received a kidney transplant, which is functioning well. Although she didn't get to Hong Kong before the take-over, she and Mitch celebrated her new kidney by taking a five-day cruise. She reports, "Everything worked out beautifully, and we had a fine time! Now we'll start planning more adventuresome trips!"

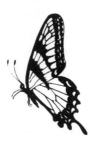

4

Rialta
I Tell My Diary My Troubles

Rialta is a lovely young Black woman who has kept a diary for years. Before lupus, her diary was filled with descriptions of activities, dates, and adolescent dreams about her future. Her lupus began ten months ago. She still writes in her diary, but now her diary tells the story of her struggle with lupus. These are excerpts:

January 12. Pain and exhaustion all the time. I've always worked extra hard, to be the best. My job was just a starting place. I was going to save money and go back to college. I really want a Ph.D. I was planning to cross out my last name, which I don't like much, and use Rialta for my last name. Dr. Rialta. I've written Dr. Rialta in this diary for two years, and now I know it's hopeless. I am lucky to have my job with the county, because the county pays my medical bills. There's no chance I'll get back to college, unless some miracle cure comes along.

June 26. Lupus is overwhelming. Today I feel so sick I can barely get out of bed. I spent the day moving from a hot bathtub to heating pads to my electric massage wand. I am so tired I have to sleep, but the pain keeps me awake. I just lie here in the most comfortable position I can find, using lots of pillows under my legs and arms. I don't dare think, because thinking and worrying are all jumbled together. I have been spilling protein in my urine, and that is always frightening. I worry that someday my kidneys may stop functioning. My lower back hurts so much that I believe I must have some sort of big infection inside my body.

I am also suffering from bowel problems. I worry that I'll have a bowel obstruction and end up with a colostomy. My doctor says that is not a part of lupus, but other doctors say it is. One thing that makes me worry is that my doctors contradict each other. To keep from worrying, I try not to think about it. This sounds crazy, but I also worry that if I think about anything awful happening, it will come true.

June 28:   How could I have told my family, just a few days ago, that I was doing well, and that my life was good? I never tell them when I am sick. I know the bad part will pass, and if I tell people how sick I am, they won't understand that I can be this sick one day and well the next. When I'm fine, they'll treat me like an invalid or just give me perplexed looks. Only people who have lupus know what it is like.

June 30. Today I feel better, and have a glimpse of hope. I stayed awake all day, and cleaned my nice, tiny apartment. Tomorrow with luck I'll be back to work.

July 1. It is wonderful to feel well. I am taking steroids again and I hate that, but now I can enjoy my life.

July 4. Hurrah! I have a date to a rock concert and dance. And I am well enough to go!

July 6. Today I am paying the price for dancing. I expected to have to spend one day in bed, resting after a day of fun, but today is the second day that I'm exhausted and in pain. I went to work anyway, because I don't want to call in sick too often, but I was totally beat. I came straight home and took a two-hour nap. Afterwards, I put gas in my car, drove to the bank to deposit my check, and had to come home to sleep again, without even shopping for tonight's dinner. I have to work tomorrow, no matter how I feel. If I quit working, what would be left for me? I am too young to spend the rest of my life doing nothing.

Mostly, I love to party. I am angry at myself for dancing and having a couple of drinks on the 4th, and that's not fair.

I'm only twenty-two years old, and I want to have a boyfriend and lead a normal life. What would become of me if I gave up? I want to have dates and dances and things.

I wish I were normal and able to do what other people do.

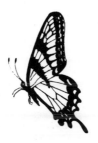

5

Nikki
I Have Chinchillas, Birds, Flowers, And My Family

I got sick very fast. It was three years ago. I always go to the rodeo every year. I was at the rodeo when my hands began to swell. I looked at my hands and I think, What is the matter with my hands? They were lumpy, they hurt. And that evening, oh my goodness, my whole body ached. I can't tell you how bad I hurt. My face had a rash.

I went to the doctor, but unfortunately my family doctor at Ft. Ord was leaving, so I had to find a different doctor. But first he gave me tests ... so many tests! So much blood! My joints ached and inside my stomach ached. I tried to explain this to the doctor, but he said all the tests were negative. Then he sent me to a rheumatologist and he told me to take Tylenol. I didn't have energy. I felt like I was carrying some kind of heavy chain. When I was standing in the kitchen, cooking, I was so tired I wanted to lie down on the floor and not get up.

Before that, oh my goodness, I had so much energy. In the old days, I worked all day cleaning offices. I owned a janitorial service. Then I came home and worked in the garden and cleaned my house and cooked and took care of my five children. I went to school to learn better English, and every Friday night my husband and I went dancing. So much energy I used to have!

I wish I had the energy to go back to school now and study more English. I love to study, and I still have some problems with the past tense. I was so worried about this interview. I thought, will I say the wrong things? I was worried because of my English. Am I saying the right things?

When I got sick, I can't do anything. And you should see what happened to my poor garden. It was ruined, because I didn't have energy to take care of it. So difficult. I kept wondering what's wrong with me, and nobody knew what was wrong. For a whole year, nobody knew.

Then I saw a new doctor, a colonel, and he read all my records and he wrote me a note. I still have the note. It says systemic lupus erythematosus. I have lupus. I never heard of such a thing. The colonel didn't want to be my doctor because he was only on temporary duty. They sent me to a psychiatrist to give me tranquilizers, but I didn't have a doctor for my lupus.

I am still trying to find a doctor. Ft. Ord doesn't have doctors any more, and I am still looking for a specialist who will take me.

I found out about our lupus group and that has helped me so much. The group has given me many friends, and that is a wonderful thing. I found other women who feel like I do. I am not crazy and I am not making up pain. The women in our lupus group understand that. I learned in the lupus group what to eat and how to take care of myself.

Lupus is very strange. The pain moves from one place to another, and I don't know why. Now I have a bad pain in my ankle, but I know some day it will be gone, and then the pain will be somewhere else.

Right now my pain isn't too bad, but I feel so tired. I'm afraid now. I'm not sure of myself any more. I want to go to the park, I want to take a bus, and then I worry, "What will happen if I get too tired and I am not at home?" I was never that way before. My goodness, I used to go everywhere. I was a fun girl. I never got sick before.

I come from the island of Hokkaido, from a little farm village. How did I meet my husband? Well, you see, I was married when I was very young. The families arranged it and I didn't even see my husband until the wedding day. We had two children, and it was a bad, bad marriage, so I found a lawyer and got a divorce. I had to do that without help from anyone in my family, even though everyone knew how bad my marriage is. In my village it is tabu to have a divorce. After a divorce, nobody wants you. I knew I could not go home to visit my family or ever again see my village. After my divorce, I lived in the city with my step-father's mistress. Her son worked on the Army base and one day he brought an American to meet me. The American was so very kind. We got married. We couldn't talk to each other, we could just smile and dance. My goodness, I can't even remember how we communicated with each other. We had some funny misunderstandings.

We have a good marriage. Deep inside of me I have my Japanese culture to help me. You know how American people are very open? Anything you want to say, you just say. But we are different. We have our pride and we don't want to hurt people, so we think before we speak. I think that made my marriage a happy one. I am so lucky.

Now my husband is sick, too. It is sad to see him sick, but now we are together. He understands my problem better, and he is very supportive. It's strange, we lupus people don't look sick, so it's hard for others to understand. My husband doesn't look so sick, but he is sick, too. The doctor told him, "Your lungs are deteriorating." I think he has emphysema. He is a house painter and that work isn't good for him, but my husband will be sixty-two soon and then he can get social security. We wait for that. We used to do very well when he had his painting business and I had my cleaning service, but lots of times he can't work and I can't work at all. What we get from the Army is enough only for our house payments.

I am fixing up my garden again, little by little. I can't be in the sun, but every day just before the sun goes down, you'll find me outside, working in my garden. Oh, and I have my four chinchillas, who are my pets, and my birds. My husband makes all my cages and he made me a special room for my plants and animals, a special room where the sun can't hurt me. Come to see my room.

(Nikki leads us into a beautiful indoor greenhouse, filled with many varieties of blooming flowers, and singing birds. The chinchillas are in large cages along one wall.) Do you like my room? So beautiful, I know it is. Every night I let my chinchillas out of their cages and they run all over this room and play with me. Oh my goodness, even though I have lupus and my husband is sick, how lucky my life is!

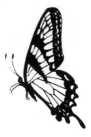

6

Dolores
Once I Was The Finest Salsa Dancer In Town

Dolores lives in a nursing home while the county tries to find a permanent facility for her thirty-year-old son, who has been a paraplegic for eleven years as a result of a gunshot wound. In spite of her lupus, Dolores took complete, twenty-four-hour-a-day care of him for over ten years, and did it so well that he hardly ever had a bed sore. She is now too ill to care for him.

Dolores: My lupus started when I went to a party and played all day in the swimming pool. I can't swim, but I liked to play in the water. That evening I was in terrible pain. I felt like I was dying. It was a burning pain, a terrible aching everywhere. I don't remember what year that was. That's when I found out I had lupus. But maybe I've always had lupus, who knows?

When I was a child, I had pains. I used to curl up in a ball, I had so much pain all over. My mother didn't believe me. She thought I was making it all up so that I wouldn't have to go to school, but I wasn't. I quit school in the sixth grade because of my pain. I was always hurting. I'd say, "Mama, I can't stand the pain." All my life it was this way.

Not all my life. I got married young, divorced, had a baby girl, and she died. The doctor said she didn't have lungs on one side, so naturally she just died. I left field work and was working in town. I didn't have money for much of anything, but I wasn't in pain for quite a while after that.

Now that I remember, I can tell you I was well then. I got married again and my husband and I had lots of good times. I had a healthy son and my husband was a good man. We both

37

worked hard, and we went to all the parties. Everybody knew that I was the best salsa and cumbia dancer in town.

When my son was nineteen years old, somebody shot him and he was totally paralyzed. I took complete care of him, even after I got lupus. Now I have lupus, anemia, diabetes, and heart trouble. I don't remember which came first.

My husband left long ago with another woman. I don't blame him. What kind of life was it, a paralyzed son and a sick wife? After he left, I found plenty of boy friends. People always liked me, because I was fun.

Now I have a new boyfriend I met at a burger stand. He's a young guy, as young as my son, and he makes me laugh. He makes me feel comfortable. He comes here to this awful place every day to visit, and he drives me to the hospital to see my son. At the hospital they take care of my son, and it takes a lot of nurses to do that. When I was at home, nobody from the county would help me with my son, even when I was so sick. Now that I am in this nursing home, he gets good care.

I don't have anything left to do in my life. I lie here and listen to the radio and sometimes I go down to the day room to talk to the nurses and ask for more morphine. I don't have strength any more. Sometimes I play bingo, but it's not much fun, because you can't win money here. Only powders and perfumes. I used to win a lot of money gambling.

When I get out of here, my boyfriend and I will go gambling. I have my own TV at home, so we'll watch TV. My boyfriend says they put me in here because I overdosed. I don't remember anything about it, but my boyfriend said I took a lot of pills. He says I wanted to kill myself. I know I was tired of being sick, and I get desperate sometimes.

Now I am on morphine all the time. It makes me restless and tired and constipated, but it takes away my pain. They give me insulin, too, for my diabetes, and I wish they'd give me something for the lupus, something that would make me better, but I haven't got a lupus doctor. Lupus doctors don't come to this nursing home. I never have gotten medicine for my lupus, and the other women in the lupus group don't understand that. Maybe it's because I am a Medicaid patient. Or is it because I'm Mexican?

They say I can never take care of my son again, so I have to let them put him in a place like this. I don't want my son in a place like this, but what can I do? After they figure out what to do with him, they'll probably send me home with my boyfriend.

I did have a lot of fun in life, once. Not when I was little and not after my son got shot and I got lupus, but in between I remember the dancing and good times. Everybody always used to say that the best thing about me was my sense of humor. I could keep everybody laughing. Now I don't find anything to laugh about.

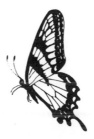

7

Maria
My Husband Is My Best Friend

Maria speaks in a hoarse whisper because of old damage to her vocal chords: My lupus started thirty years ago. When it started, Stan and I had been married eight years and our son, Timmy, was four years old. I'd gotten a sunburn the day before, playing tennis. Suddenly every joint in my body hurt, especially in my hands and fingers, and I had a rash.

Stan: I told her to call the doctor. When she phoned him, she only told him about the rash on her face. I said, "Tell him about your hands."

Maria: I was most interested in the rash on my face. (She giggles.) It was ugly. Well, the doctor had just gotten back from his vacation. He always read his medical journals while he was on vacation, and he'd read about the rash. So, when he saw me, he sent me to the hospital for a blood test and he called back in two hours and said I had an appointment at Stanford University hospital the next day. I got my diagnosis right away: systemic lupus erythematosus. It didn't mean a thing to me.

Stan: When she was diagnosed, she was one of only forty-nine known cases in California. There must have been lots more that weren't identified.

Maria: I tried to keep on working. I was a secretary for a realtor. I could hardly walk from my desk to the back of the office, and walking up and down the stairs was agony. I was diagnosed in August and I kept working until December. I had to quit then, because I couldn't do the work.

Nobody had heard of lupus. The doctors put me on massive doses of aspirin, but I kept getting worse. They didn't know I should avoid the sun, so I would lie in the sun whenever I had time off. I love the sun and I love to swim.

Stan: The doctors told her not to quit working, because they were afraid she'd lie in bed all day. They said she'd have to keep moving her joints or they would freeze. It turned out not to be true for lupus.

I asked the doctor what was going to happen to Maria, and he said she would live five to five-and-a-half years. I couldn't tell Maria. There was no one I could tell. Back then, I thought doctors were gods. I was desolate, in terrible emotional pain, believing I was going to lose her, and there was no one I could talk to. It was the worst time of my life, those five years, waiting for her to die.

Maria: They never told me I was supposed to die in five years. If they'd told me, I might have done it. That's how much I believed doctors. Since I didn't know what was going on in me, I wasn't scared. I'm not a worrier. I just live from day to day. I still don't worry. Stan worries for both of us.

Sometimes the pain was so bad that I couldn't turn over in bed, and when Stan turned over it was agony. I asked the doctor what to do, and he said to buy twin beds. I told him I didn't get married to sleep in a twin bed. So we got a king-size bed instead, and that was better. But I kept getting worse. I was in and out of the hospital.

Stan: Almost exactly five years from the day she was diagnosed, she went back into the hospital at Stanford for two months. She was down to ninety pounds and was just shrivelling away. I assumed she was dying, like the doctor predicted. Then they started her on Prednisone and Cytoxan, and that turned it around.

Maria: I met a nurse at Stanford who helped me a lot. She had lupus, too. She taught me how to live with pain and how to react to doctors. She taught me to stop being so cooperative. Before that, I let them do three bone marrow tests, and other terrible tests which I didn't need, because they were doing research on lupus. I didn't know I could refuse.

After that, I went into remission. It was wonderful! I came home from the hospital well and happy, and that was when I got kicked out by one of the specialists. He told me, since I no longer had any symptoms of lupus, I could go in the sun if I wanted to.

Stan: And I said, "No, you can't go in the sun." She was so excited, I felt awful telling her this, but I didn't want her to risk getting sick again. She went back to the doctor for a checkup, and he asked her, "How was the sun?" And she said ...

Maria: I told the doctor that I didn't go in the sun because my husband said not to. The doctor said, "Who are you going to believe about your disease, me or your husband?" And I said, "Well, I've had my husband longer than I've had you, so I guess I'll believe him." Then he said, "In that case, you don't need ME any more." And that was the end of my seeing him.

Stan: A couple of weeks later she got a phone call from the doctor. He said he was sorry, and he would continue to see her. By then I had found another specialist for her.

Maria: I told that doctor, "I don't need YOU any more."

Stan: And there was another doctor who told her that her worst problem was depression.

Maria: I have depression on and off, but it's not my worst problem.

Stan: Even after the five years were up, I kept expecting Maria to die. If I hadn't been told that she would die, we would have had a much better time of it.

Maria: We had fun, Stan. It wasn't all bad. Remember when Tim was playing baseball? I wore a big hat and long sleeves and gloves, and we went to every game.

Stan: We had fun. But I was in agony all those years for nothing.

Maria: Thank God Stan never told me until years later.

Stan: I'm not worried any more. I think Maria will probably outlive me. (Chuckles.)

Maria: No, I think we'll go together.

Stan: You asked how we coped during the sick times? We had help. Maria's parents bought us the house next door to theirs, so they could help take care of Maria and Tim. Still, there were lots of difficult times. Do you mind if I tell about ... you know?

Maria: Go ahead.

Stan: Well, once when she got home from the hospital - - she was on massive doses of prednisone - - she developed a psychosis. She wasn't logical, she wasn't rational. For instance, Maria always managed our money, so one day I said we'd have to be careful about money now, because we'd had some big expenses. The next month I found out she hadn't paid any bills at all. She was being careful by keeping all our money in the bank.

And then one day she began to dye everything cardinal red.

Maria: I wanted everything cheerful, and red was the most cheerful color. (Laughs.) I don't remember much. It was a blank period.

Stan: She dyed our drapes red and then she sent me out to buy more dye. I didn't know what to do. I drove around for awhile, thinking, and then I came back and told her there was no more red dye in the whole town. I telephoned the doctor at Stanford and told him what was happening. He said, "Yeah, that's steroid psychosis." I asked him if it would be all right to tell her what was happening and why, and he said, "Say anything you want, but don't expect that she'll listen to you."

I thought it was worth a try. I sat her down and told her that she had this steroid psychosis. "You're not rational right now. You're doing things that are not normal for you. It's due to the medication." I told her, "I want you to listen to me, and we'll get through this." And she did.

Maria: I've always trusted Stan. We've made it this far because we trust each other.

Stan: A lot of couples split up when they have troubles, sickness. It seemed to make us stronger. It's kind of funny - - when she was down, I was up, and then one day, when she was in remission, my back gave out. I had back surgery and my doctor told me I couldn't continue doing physical labor. I asked what I could do, and he recommended my new career. I got books and pamphlets and read about it, and I liked the idea. I was in a position where I could go to school, so I went to school for three years and got a very good job. Sometimes I think the back did me a favor.

Maria: I took care of him when he had surgery. We hung in there. And our son was very good. He was a thoughtful person. Like, one day he wanted to go somewhere, but he said, "I can't go, because you're sick." I told him to go. "We are not going to hold you up, ever." So he went and had a good time, but he was thoughtful that way.

I was in remission for eleven years, and then I had another flare. That's when I lost my voice. I had seizures and respiratory arrest, and my vocal chords were damaged when I was intubated. They tried to fix my voice, but couldn't.

Stan: Her vocal chords are frozen. She can't really use them at all.

Maria: I had speech therapy. At first, no one could hear me, but now they can. I've gotten to be afraid of crowds, because if anything goes wrong, I can't yell. It's frightening to go through life whispering.

I was an outdoor person who enjoyed the sun and swimming, but now I have indoor hobbies. I'll show you my ceramics. Stan helps me when my hands are too sore to do tiny work. Besides my ceramics, I spend a lot of time reading. I read everything I can get my hands on. It doesn't matter what kind of book, fiction, non-fiction, I just love to read. People give me books, and sometimes when I feel well enough, I go to the library to choose my own.

Stan and I are very religious. We have lots of friends at our church, and when I am too sick to go to church, a friend brings me Holy Communion.

I can't clean our house any more. Nowadays, I usually sleep until noon, and I take a nap in the afternoon, but I do get fixed up for Stan. That nurse at Stanford, long ago, taught me that no matter how you feel, you should get dressed and put on make-up every day. So in the afternoon after my nap, I take a shower and then I sit down and rest. Then I comb my hair and get dressed up. I want to look the best I can when Stan comes home.

Stan: We have a good life. In the past, we never used to plan to do anything, because we weren't sure we had a future. Now we plan whatever we want. Then, if we can do it, fine. If not, we'll do it another time.

Maria: Last month we drove to Arizona to visit our son and daughter-in-law and our grandchildren.

Stan: Our long-term plan right now is to buy a truck and a trailer, and travel. I've worked long enough to have plenty of vacation time.

Maria: After my parents both died, we bought this new house and we're still fixing it up. We live on the first floor, and there is plenty of room for Tim and his family upstairs, when they come to visit. Stan and I have been together thirty-six years now. He is still my best friend.

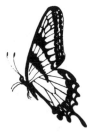

8

Joyce
I Am A Survivor

You could say that my lupus started with a bang! I was healthy, happy, newly married, had a good job, and within two months of our honeymoon I was temporarily a quadriplegic. I got lupus poly-myelitis and was unable to move. Art, my new husband, had to dress me, brush my teeth, do everything for me. I couldn't even open my own mouth.

I began to be able to function little by little. To get out of bed, I'd grab the top of my head by the hair and lift and turn. I would sit on the rocking chair with my underpants on the floor next to me. I'd work to get my feet into them and finally after a lot of effort, I'd be able to tug them up to my knees. To do this, I'd have to take hold of one hand and push it into the panties, try to grab a piece of the material, and then pull up on that hand with my other hand. It was very difficult. My goal for the day was to dress myself.

I loved that big rocking chair, because it was the safest place for me. When I would start to choke, I'd rock myself forward as hard as I could, and throw myself on the floor. That would jar the phlegm loose in my throat so that I could spit and breathe. It was a crazy, terrible time, but I survived.

My tooth brushing was funny. I'd squeeze the toothpaste and then I'd find out where it went. I'd put my toothbrush on the blob of paste, wherever it had landed, and I'd try to brush my teeth.

When I did something new, I'd be so excited, I'd call my Mom and say, "You'll never believe what I just did." And then I'd tell her, "I put on my blouse by myself," or "I got up the stairs without any help."

The first six months were really bad. Sometimes I felt like giving up, but I'm the kind of person who says, OK, I will learn how to deal with this. And my husband is the same. He stuck with me in spite of everything.

One reason I did well was that my husband didn't help me unless I really needed it. He knew that if I wanted to do something badly enough I'd learn how to do it.

For instance, as soon as I could walk to the garage, I stole my car. I got my hands under the steering wheel, put the car into reverse, picked up my leg, and put it on the gas pedal. When I got the car into the street, I put my hand under the steering wheel again and got it in the drive position, and then I drove down the country roads by myself. I never thought about how dangerous or stupid this was. When I got home, there was my husband waiting for me, speechless. I couldn't get the car into park, so he had to jump across me to do it.

He sold the car for me, and bought me an automatic with the controls down where I could maneuver them with one hand.

Before the first year was up, my colon perforated and I had to have a colostomy. I had these terrible craters in my front, because my fistulas didn't heal. I had major wounds below my navel that were so wide that I could lay a bar of soap in them.

As I walked to bed we'd hear this loud fart-like sound from the colostomy bag. And sometimes at night I'd roll over in my sleep and the bag would be knocked off, and my husband would say, "Honey, you'd better wake up."

I'd say, "What's the matter?"

"I think you shit the bed."

Things like that. My hands would be swollen and sore, and lots of times I couldn't make my fingers work. He would have to cut the little stupid thing on the bag for me. It was demeaning.

When the fistulas were finally healed and the surgeon sewed me up again, my husband said he couldn't tell if I was coming or going, because my front side had two big butts just like my back side. We laughed about it, because laughing feels better than crying.

I had another perforation ten years later. My husband had just finished working a double shift, and was so exhausted that I couldn't get him to wake up. I said, "Honey, I'm in pain," and he didn't respond. I was furious that he wouldn't wake up, so I got myself downstairs and into the car, put it into cruise control, and bopped myself to the hospital. I walked into the emergency room and told them, "I have a perforated colon."

I showed the emergency-room doctor where I felt the tear in my abdomen, and he said, "First we'll order some tests."

I said, "Yes, I know, blood, urine, Xrays, and they aren't going to show anything. I've been through this before." I was trying to be calm. The last time I was in this hospital I had a perforated colon, so I know what is going on inside me. That time I was here nine days, while you guys said nothing was wrong with me. This time you are going to listen to me!" I told him to call my surgeon and my doctor immediately. "I am in a lot of pain, so hurry."

He wanted at the very least to perform a colonoscopy.

I said, "Do a CAT scan and you'll see it is perforated. A colonoscopy will make the perforation worse." I knew, and he didn't, what was wrong with me.

Then I started to scream, "It's tearing more." He gave me morphine, did the CAT scan, and minutes later reported, "You've got a perforation and there's gas in your abdomen."

I said, "No kidding."

My surgeon arrived. Just before I was wheeled into surgery, I phoned home. My husband said, "Where the hell are you?"

I said, "In the hospital, honey. You better come on down."

The next day my doctor thanked me for hanging tough and not letting them do a colonoscopy or waste time with lab work.

He said that the reason I was alive was that I knew my own body and was insistent on the correct treatment.

While I was in the hospital, I started going to our lupus group. Claudia Pagano was my nurse, and she wheeled me to the meetings from my hospital bed. I'd go in my hospital gown with my IV attached, and I'd laugh and joke with the other women. They kept me wanting to live in spite of those bad times.

I wasn't allowed to eat. I lived almost a year on intravenous feedings without eating anything, so that my bowel could heal. I cooked dinner for the family and went out to lunch with my girlfriends without eating, and it was OK. I wanted to be well, and this was what I had to do.

Since then I have been well, more or less, except for the lupus pain. When you've had a perforated ulcer, you can't take anti-inflammatories, which is difficult. At night, if the pain is too bad, I watch old comedies or reruns of the Mary Tyler Moore shows. One of my hobbies is genealogy, and I work on it at night when I can't sleep.

My days are kind of chaotic. I visit my mother and an ex-neighbor, who are in nursing homes now. I take care of my dogs and cats. I go to garage sales and second-hand stores to search for interesting odds and ends.

I like to refinish old furniture. I'll buy a piece, strip it, finish it, and then sometimes I'll keep it and sometimes I'll sell it. That lovely old church bench over there, for instance, took me weeks of sanding and polishing, and I'll probably end up selling it. I decorate these wooden boxes, which I call "memory-makers," because people buy them to hold their personal treasures. I make and frame collages of old photos, lace, and whatever I choose. I do woodburning, the way it was done a century ago. Because of the pain in my hands, I work slowly. Lots of people come here to see my home and all the things I have for sale.

I regret having had to give up my work outside my home, especially my last job, managing an animal hospital, but I like what I'm still able to create here at home.

I'm not a super religious person. I believe in God. I believe each step you have to take is a step up. I have this statue of Peter and Jesus that my uncle gave me, and whenever I think I can't keep going, I look at it.

Yes, I am proud of the way I manage my life. I had a lot of support and I think I have a talent for living. And I have a sense of humor.

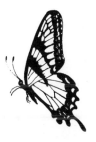

9

Vera
One Day I Lost My Memory

Sickness has been a big part of my life. When I was a child
I was always sick—with tonsillitis, before there was peni-
cillin, and so much stomach trouble. Every day, I'd drink milk
and afterwards I'd vomit. My stomach was always hurting.
We lived on a farm, and used to sell our corn at a roadside
stand. After picking the corn, I couldn't go to the stand to sell
it, even though I wanted to be there. I always had to take a nap.
Sometimes, my legs would puff up and I'd get the chills, and
be so tired I could hardly walk. I think I had lupus even then.
From my earliest days, I would get sick from the sun and from
milk, but, of course, no one figured out what was wrong.

When I started going to doctors as an adult, I found out my
chemistry was out of balance. Sometimes my blood pressure
was low and another time it was high. Sometimes my thyroid
was low and then again it might be high. My system had gone
bananas. I began having severe colitis.

I spent years telling doctors how tired I was. They didn't
know what was wrong, so they kept giving me different medicines. At work, I'd sit all day at my desk without moving around
much, because I honestly was too tired to walk. They thought
I was dedicated to my job, and I got raises, but the truth was I
was too tired to move.

Then one day I lost my memory. I couldn't remember how
to process the computer I'd been running for several years. I
felt as if a blank wall had come down, separating me from everything I ever knew. I couldn't remember how to do anything
in the office. My husband and I loved to play Scrabble, and I
couldn't play any more. I couldn't put words together. When I

talked with people, I would lose my train of thought and not have any idea what I had been saying. I was terrified and humiliated.

I quit my job without telling anyone what was wrong. I didn't know what else to do. I had lots of sick leave and compensation time, but I wasn't thinking clearly enough to remember this. When I quit, I lost all the money and retirement benefits I was entitled to receive.

The doctors discovered that I had lupus. I had never heard of lupus before, but as soon as I could think clearly again, I began to study the disease.

I go to public lectures on lupus and I learn everything I can. I know a lot about the disease. I even keep track of the newest ways of treating symptoms I have never had. You might say that lupus is my hobby as well as my disease. I joined the lupus foundation and I love our lupus support group.

When I got ulcerative colitis, I joined that organization, too. I watch my diet, read everything about these two diseases, and do everything the literature suggests. Now my colitis is healed. Also, I have no memory problems any more.

The doctor thinks I may have some heart problems, so I am studying about that now.

Lupus is annoying and painful. One minute you feel horrible and then the next day you are fine. I have days without pain, and that is lucky. When I get tired, I lie down. I can listen to my body now that I know what's wrong.

I work in my garden late in the afternoon, even though I always have to take a nap afterwards. I do volunteer work for a charitable organization that raises money to help disabled children. I don't want to be useless.

I think all of the people in our lupus group look for things to do for other people. I don't know if they told you that, but they are all good people who care about others. When you are helping other people, you don't have as much time to worry about yourself.

I'm a worrier. I worry about getting things done. For example, right now I am worrying about getting my Christmas cards done on time. I send over 100 Christmas cards every year, and I enjoy writing notes on each one, but I would feel guilty if I didn't get all of them done on time. It's a big chore, especially when my hands are hurting.

Faith helps me. If you have faith you can accept what happens to you. Some people feel that God causes their problems because "He doesn't like me," or "I did something wrong." I don't think that way. I have a feeling that is hard to explain. It's a feeling - - God is taking care of all of us, and we will be all right in His Hands.

I don't let myself get down in the dumps. After all, isn't it bad enough to have lupus without being depressed or angry about it?

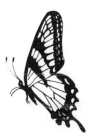

10

Louise
Lupus Cost Me My Marriage

Before lupus, I had a normal, happy life. We lived in Dallas. I was married, had two young sons, and we were a close, loving family. My husband and I both worked. In addition to my work, I was active in our church and the PTA. We were members of one of the best golf and tennis clubs in our area. Every year, we went on a luxury cruise, paid for by my husband's company. I was beautiful then, I really was, and my husband was proud of me.

Then, suddenly, I was ill. I hurt in every joint in my body, had a rash, and was so tired I couldn't get out of bed. I thought it was a new kind flu, but it persisted. I went to a doctor, who hospitalized me and did a lot of tests. He said, "You have lupus, but don't worry. It's only a mild case."

I went back to work, determined not to let lupus get me down. In addition to my full-time job, I became president of the PTA and room mother in my children's school, while I was so tired and swollen and full of pain that I could barely endure my life. I hid my pain from the family, and when it was too bad I'd lock myself in the bedroom and cry. I had high blood pressure and sometimes had difficulty breathing, but I believed I could conquer it all by will power, working extra hard, and trusting in God.

Because I hid my misery from my family, none of them understood what I was going through. My husband complained when I couldn't go to dances at the country club, because it was important to his work that he be seen there with me. Once, when I just couldn't move, I told my younger son, "I'm tired, I have to lie down." He said, "Why can't you be like the other mothers?" After that, I tried harder to hide my pain.

I began having urinary tract infections, kidney stones, and my high blood pressure was dangerously high. I was very swollen. My physician referred me to a nephrologist, who told me, "Your kidneys are functioning, but not well." He tried chemotherapy to save the kidneys, but all it did was made me loose my hair. I became more and more ill.

One morning right after Christmas, I was having increasing difficulty breathing, so I drove myself to the emergency room. Naturally, I drove myself - - I was still trying to pretend I could do anything.

They rushed me into ICU, the intensive care unit of the hospital, and everything began happening fast. They were trying to put a tube down the artery in my neck, because my kidneys had failed and my lungs were full of fluid. Lots of doctors and nurses were involved. I was terrified. I was tilted with my head down, so I couldn't breathe. They had this sheet over me so I wouldn't see what they were doing, and the problem was that they couldn't see me, either. I couldn't breathe and I couldn't get their attention. I was choking to death. Finally, I was able to grab a doctor's arm and pinch as hard as I could. I wouldn't let go. He looked at me and saw my distress.

He yelled, "Get her up, get her up right now." I was suffocating and drowning, and finally they sat me up and I could breathe again.

Then someone said, "We'll have to start all over again." After all this torture, they wanted to try again to get the dialysis working in my neck.

I fought them. I wouldn't let them do it. Finally they went into my thigh instead.

Dialysis is terrible. You can smell the stuff, a mixture of blood and I don't know what. It was awful and I was gagging. I can't tell you how awful it was. When I complained, they told me I was going to have to have this done all the rest of my life. I hadn't known that, or understood. They were going to do this horrible thing to me, over and over again.

They insisted that I would have to have the dialysis tube in my neck, and I said "No." They argued with me for three or four hours, I think. The doctor said, "It will be easier this time, because we've already dialyzed you once, and also the fluid is mostly gone from your lungs. It'll be OK this time." But I wouldn't let anyone touch me. I said, "Find me a different doctor."

Because I insisted, a new doctor came in, who stayed right next to me, so that I could see him, and he got it into me much quicker and he kept talking to me, telling me what he was doing, and this time it was OK. It wasn't fine, but I wasn't totally panicked.

After a month of this type of dialysis, they said I could dialyze myself at home. Thank God for that! Some people don't have difficulty with hospital dialysis, but I did. Perhaps my problem was emotional, because of that terrible first time.

I was on dialysis for two years. During the first year of dialysis at home, after I got my strength back, I continued trying to prove that nothing could conquer me. I went back to work and continued all my activities. Although we hired a cleaning person twice a week at home, I'd clean before she came. I still wanted to pretend to be in charge of my family, my life, everything.

The second year, I was so sick and depressed that I couldn't pretend any longer. I stopped being president of the PTA. I stopped my volunteer work. I was too ugly to be seen at the country club. I had to quit my job. That's when our family began to fall apart.

I was no fun to be with. I think I behaved like Jekyll and Hyde. You know how it is when you have a really bad headache, and people keep asking you to do things for them. All you want is to be left alone. That's how it was for me. I hurt so much. My whole body ached. I couldn't help anyone. I wanted to scream, "Please, someone, do something for me!" But there was no one to help me. I became more depressed. Probably I had been depressed since the beginning of my lupus, but up to that second year I was able to hide my weaknesses.

And then, out of the blue, I'd have a couple of good days and I'd feel as if I could do anything for anybody. Nobody understood this. They'd say, "How come you feel good today, but yesterday, when I wanted your help, you said you were too sick to help me?" Well, that's exactly how lupus is, even though families don't understand.

My home life got - - broken. That's the only word that fits. My husband found another woman. I wasn't beautiful and I couldn't go places with him. My figure was gone, and I didn't want sex. The woman he was used to, who could do anything, who was beautiful and sexy, no longer existed. Lupus killed that woman.

That's why I say that lupus destroyed our family.

Peritonitis set in from my dialysis, and while I was in the hospital, he asked for a divorce and left. My children and I moved to California to be near my sisters. They do help me as much as they can.

After more than two years on dialysis I received a kidney transplant. For six months it was hell because of problems with rejection, but since then I've been fine. I mean, I still have my lupus problems, but not the problems with the transplant. With Prednisone I've gained thirty pounds, and I hate that. When I am fat, I consider myself a failure as a woman.

On the positive side, I've made wonderful friends in our lupus group. We've taught each other to care about ourselves. I spent my life taking care of everybody else. I put myself last. Now, I am learning to put myself first.

I have good days and bad days, and on the good days I am doing things for me. I'm taking better care of my body and I am not depressed, the way I was before. Yoga is wonderful! I have two yoga classes a week, and after the class I have lunch with some of the other participants.

Last month I took a vacation to Reno with my sisters. We gambled and enjoyed the floor shows. It's not the same as the Caribbean cruises, but I had a happy time. My children are older now, and pretty much on their own.

I think I deserve to feel proud of myself, just because I still exist. I didn't kill myself or drown in my own self-pity. I don't know what the future may bring, but I will find a way to take good care of myself and ask for help when I need it.

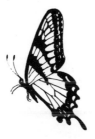

11

Beth
My Doctor Said I Was A Hypochondriac

I was thirty-seven years old when I was diagnosed with lupus, but I think it started long before that. From the time I was twenty-five, I had intermittent shoulder and back pain, fatigue, and chronic diarrhea. I remember that I slept while car-pooling to work mornings, and would arrive feeling useless and unable to think. Often I ended in the boss' office in tears simply because I was so tired. I found out that I was lactose intolerant, and the rest of my symptoms were chalked up to stress. I did feel better when I gave up all dairy products, stopped working, and stayed home with my two young children.

After a year I had to go to work again for financial reasons. I didn't go back to my 8 to 5 office job. Instead, in order to be at home when my children needed me, I began cleaning model homes and offices at night. I didn't want to make a career of this, so, with my family's encouragement, I enrolled in graduate school. At that time I must have been in remission, because I earned excellent grades, cared for my children, and continued my cleaning work. Whenever I had free time, I loved to lie in the sun. It made me feel sleepy and relaxed, as if I'd had a glass or two of fine wine.

All of a sudden, I began having allergy symptoms, and I became more and more exhausted, but I didn't have health insurance, so I couldn't afford to see a physician. I assured myself that I was just getting older, working too hard, and under too much stress. It wasn't easy going to school and raising children, as I could only study when they were asleep.

They seemed to be quite casual about my illness. Through a fog of sleep I'd hear one or the other introduce me to new school friends. "Brenda, this is my mother. She sleeps a lot." They talked to me while I was asleep, asking to invite friends to spend the night or, sometimes, wondering if we were going to have dinner. Later, when I was awake they'd repeat their messages and tell the answers I'd given in my sleep. They didn't worry. I'd been like this as long as they could remember, so they took my behavior for granted.

Finally, I felt so sick that I went to the student health clinic, where the doctor said I must have allergies. He refused to treat me until I was willing to get rid of my hamsters, dogs, and birds, which I wouldn't do because I had no reason to believe they were causing my problems. I think that was his way of getting rid of me.

When I received my degree, I was offered a very good job, with good health insurance. As soon as I was eligible for medical care, I saw an allergist, who tested me and said that he had never seen anyone who was allergic to so many things. I seemed to be allergic to everything that grew in the ground or landed on it, including plants and trees, mold, vegetables, grass, and seeds.

I was not allergic to pet hair or pet dandruff. There would be no more death mandates against my pets, who were growing older but were still with me!

The doctor began treating my allergies and those symptoms disappeared, but I continued to be fatigued, so he took a blood test, and told me that I might have lupus because my ANA titer was 1:1400 (the normal range was less than 1:40.) I had never heard of lupus.

He said it was a disease like arthritis, with rashes from exposure to the sun. I assured him that I couldn't have lupus, because my children and I spent every weekend in the sun, and I never had a rash. He sent me to a rheumatologist.

The rheumatologist told me, "You have nothing to worry about. You don't have lupus."

I continued the shots to desensitize my immune system against all my allergies, and was grimly determined to mini-mize the importance of my exhaustion. I told myself that ev-eryone was tired from time to time, and I shouldn't baby myself. Whenever I felt well, I bicycled all over the countryside with my son, taught my children to swim, lifted weights at a local health club during lunch hours, and, of course, lay in the sun. I became more and more fatigued.

I began getting severe sunburns after only brief exposure to the sun. On a camping trip with my children and friends, I lay in the sun for only ten minutes, became sleepy, and went inside a tent to nap. When I woke up, I had a rash all over the inside of my legs and arms. It burned intensely, like poison oak, and every joint in my body seemed to ache. I'd forgotten about lupus, and thought I was having an allergic reaction to the trees. My body was burning, and I became nauseated and short of breath. I became very depressed, as I told myself that I would never again be able to enjoy nature and camping.

After using antihistamines and calamine lotion, the burn-ing and shortness of breath lessened somewhat, although I re-mained too weak to hike. In spite of every proof to the contrary, I didn't let myself believe that the sun could cause such prob-lems. A week later I went with my children to a swimming pool. I didn't feel well enough to swim, so I was fully dressed in slacks and a V-neck shirt, as I sat by the pool. In just a few minutes, I got a terrible sunburn on my neck, and developed welts. This time I went to a dermatologist, who biopsied the welts on my neck and told me I had systemic lupus erythema-tosus.

He referred me back to the rheumatologist, who said sar-castically, "Sure, now that you know what the symptoms are, you've managed to develop the right symptoms." He laughed at me.

Throughout my adult years, when I was so often exhausted and hurting, I told myself that I must be a hypochondriac, and now a physician was making the same diagnosis! I was humiliated.

I was also angry enough to choose a different rheumatologist, who made a definitive diagnosis of SLE based on my symptoms and history (joint pains, fatigue, and depression), a positive ANA, LE, anti-SM, and a false positive syphilis test. By the time the lab tests came back, I had the characteristic butterfly rash on my nose and cheeks. There was no doubt at all about my diagnosis.

He also diagnosed Hirshimoto thyroiditis, which is an autoimmune disease caused by antibodies attacking the thyroid. This condition would have to be monitored and in the future I might need thyroid replacement medication. An ophthalmologist diagnosed Sjogren's syndrome, which is experienced as dry mouth and eyes, and is treated with "artificial tears."

The rheumatologist explained that it is common with lupus to have other overlapping autoimmune diseases. Neither Hirshimoto thyroiditis or Sjogren's disease cause serious consequences. What was serious was the lupus itself. The rheumatologist gave me injections of Depomedrol (a long-lasting steroid) and ACTH to stimulate my adrenal glands. He prescribed Trillisate, an NSAID; Plaquenil, an anti-malarial drug: and Prozac, an anti-depressant.

At first I resisted taking Prozac, and told the rheumatologist that everything in my life was great except for the lupus, so I certainly didn't need drugs for depression. I loved my job, my children, my home, and my friends. I think that I discounted my depression, because I didn't want to be considered a "psych case." The doctor convinced me that depression can be chemically based and is very common with lupus, so I took the Prozac.

I felt better, but continued to have severe joint pains, because for me Trillisate was ineffective. The doctor prescribed

Naprosyn and Feldene, also non-steroids, and they worked better for me.

The steroid injections gave me intermittent and inconsistent relief, so I switched to Prednisone, which gives quick relief from pain and other symptoms, but has had annoying side effects, such as weight gain. I experimented until I found a regime that fits for me. I begin a course of Prednisone whenever I have a flare, which is about three or four times a year: 20 milligrams of Prednisone daily for two weeks; 15 milligrams daily for one week; 10 milligrams daily for one week; 5 milligrams daily for one or two weeks. I make the changes in dosage on Saturdays, when I have two days for resting, and I try to afford a massage on those Saturdays. My rheumatologist believes in my ability to make my own schedule, depending on what my body tells me. I appreciate him very much for this. In addition, he's a good person, who cares about his patients and keeps up on the latest lupus research.

I can't bicycle any more, and sometimes I hurt too much to enjoy walking. However, two winters ago I was able to go to the mountains to ski for the first time in my life. It was wonderful! I endure the hard times in my illness by keeping in mind that I will feel good and have fun again.

When I can't get to sleep because my joints hurt, I get out of bed and do yoga stretching positions. It takes away the pain. I go to sleep more quickly and sleep more soundly.

Whenever I am outside, I wear clothing that covers me fully, including a long-sleeved shirt, long pants, gloves, hat, and sunglasses. Although they are not very stylish, I buy my clothes from the Sun Precautions catalog (1-800-882-7860), because the clothes are especially made for their sun-protective qualities. Even with these clothes, I use sunscreen every time I leave the house, whether or not the sun is shining.

I work Mondays and Tuesdays at the office, take Wednesdays at home, and then go back to the office on Thursdays and

Fridays. For me this is an ideal schedule, because I can't work effectively more than two days at a stretch without a day of rest in between.

At work, I make my life as easy as possible, by avoiding stress. I refuse overtime, don't volunteer for extra-curricular meetings or get involved with people who are emotionally draining. I have explained to everyone at work exactly what is wrong with me. I don't deny my pain or pretend I can do things that hurt me. I keep careful track of what is going on inside my body and try to figure out accurately what causes increased pain or flares. For example, I discovered that the halogen light over my desk was giving me trouble, so I asked that it be replaced with a different kind of lighting. Everyone understands my need for an easy schedule and makes allowances when I sometimes have to nap after lunch.

On Wednesdays I keep a very easy but productive schedule. I sleep an extra hour in the morning, because I don't have to fight commute traffic. I am usually most stiff and sore in the morning, so after breakfast I sit in a hot bath while I read reports and answer business phone calls. Then I am ready to work at my computer for an hour or two. I have a late lunch and, after lunch, nap before going back to my computer.

I have cut down on housework and all non-essential activities. After dusk I love to garden, and my biggest luxury is my gardener, whom I hire once a month to do all the heavy work. My garden is filled with flowers, vegetables, and small fruit trees.

My children are in their teens now, and usually are enjoyable. On work days, we exist on take-out food, which they much prefer to having to help me cook. Although I am an expert on the avoidance of stress at work, home is another matter. There are times when I have to put up with screaming quarrels, sobs, and other teenage drama, but we also laugh a lot and have fun together. I remember my own youth and know that by comparison my son and daughter are doing very well. Whenever I can't stand the uproar, I tell them "I am taking time out," and go to my room. They don't seem to worry about my illness, perhaps because they are used to it by now. From the time I was diagnosed, I've told them everything I know about lupus and assured them that my lupus is not life-threatening.

Once my daughter was certain that she had caught it from me. "I have lupus, too," she announced as she collapsed on the couch. But most of the time, she's too busy with her school and love life to consider herself ill.

At present I have no man in my life. I am looking for someone who is interesting, lovable, and doesn't object to a partner who is ill a lot.

Although I've experimented with lots of different pain relievers in the past few years, nothing relieves joint pain and fatigue as much as massage therapy and acupuncture. These treatments are not covered by my insurance, so I don't get acupuncture any more, and have to limit my massage to the weeks when I am getting off steroids. I think it is an injustice that insurance companies will not cover these forms of treatment, that alleviate pain and suffering, but will pay for narcotics that keep people sedated without bringing relief.

I gain so much, more than I can describe, from my lupus support group, just from knowing and talking to others who have experienced some of the same problems I have.

Everyone in our group wonders what in their past may have contributed to their having lupus. The question often asked is, "Why did I get lupus?" In my case, I believe that there may be a connection between having a chronic viral illness and developing an autoimmune disorder.

I contracted herpes when I was eighteen years old, before there was any treatment or cure for it. My immune system must have recognized that a virus had invaded my system and organized a response to the virus. The unsuccessful attempt to

develop antibodies, against the herpes virus, may have intensi-
fied into an attack against my own cells. After I became ill
with lupus, my herpes dramatically disappeared in spite of the
fact that I continued to have stress, fevers, and other problems
that in the past would have precipitated an outbreak of herpes.

My doctors say that they have seen no research linking herpes and lupus, but in our group we continue to discuss possible
connections between diseases, as well as hereditary factors.

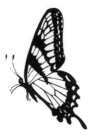

12

Meg
It Is A Challenge To Live On $660 A Month

I contracted lupus ten years ago, when I was fifty-eight. I knew something had gone wrong when I couldn't make it up the stairs to my third-floor apartment. Within a few days, I had terrible pain in my joints, difficulty breathing, and a very unusual fatigue. The fatigue is indescribable. I was working full time and had always been a high-energy person, and now I felt incapable of getting out of bed.

The doctor tried to slough me off, saying I should rest more, but I wouldn't let him ignore me. He ordered dozens of tests, and all were negative. I told him, "No matter what the tests say, there is something very wrong in my body. I want you to find out what it is." Finally, he said, "As a last resort, we'll test for lupus, but it's a disease of child-bearing years." The tests were positive.

I could no longer work, and soon my money was gone. I was declared disabled and put on SSI, (Supplementary Security Income). Without it, I would have starved to death. I have public housing now, one room with a kitchenette, and I manage on $660 a month. It is a challenge. I can't go on social security, although I am eligible for $1400 a month, because then I would be ineligible for Medicaid. My medicine costs over $1000 a month.

I was doing pretty well until two years ago, when I had the strokes that left me legally blind and partially paralyzed on my right side. One kidney has failed, but the other carries on, thank heavens. I don't have family, so I have to figure out for myself how to keep going. The county sends a woman to my apartment two hours a day, five days a week, to cook and clean for me, and the blind society sends me talking books. Unfortunately, they have a poor selection. I order books I want, and they send me what they have.

I keep busy. I work with Senior Action Network, a good group of people who care about local social issues, like problems with buses, taxicabs, all the issues that are vital to those of us who are disabled. I like to picket in my wheelchair with this group, but I have trouble getting to picket lines. I am allowed to buy $60 in taxi scripts each month for only $6, and I have to be very careful to make them last all month.

Unfortunately, the bus line that goes by my apartment has no buses for those of us with handicaps. It's a wonderful line that goes everywhere I need to go, but I can't use it. The step is too high. So I ration my taxi rides to the trips that are most important to me.

In spite of talking books, it is difficult to get used to a life without reading. I attend classes regularly in a senior enrichment program on campus. All sorts of subjects are taught, philosophy, ethics, poetry writing, and psychology, for example. I asked for and received a scholarship, so I don't have to pay for these courses. Usually I attend classes without being able to read the assigned books. I just spent $25 for the audio-book of **Sophie's World,** because it was the only book assigned for that beginning philosophy course. I love the book and have listened to it over and over, but I won't be able to afford $25 again for a long time. That was a big splurge. I am very pleased with these courses and feel like a kid, as I figure out what I'll be taking next.

I do a lot of interesting things. Even though I can't see much, I still love to go to museums. Often, I am given two free concert tickets to the symphony, and I bribe an acquaintance to drive me there, in exchange for a free ticket.

The most embittering part of being ill is that I have lost my old friends. They deserted me. I would not have believed this possible. Before lupus, I had lots of friends, and we partied and did all sorts of fun things together. As soon as I got lupus, they began to avoid me. And now that I am quite incapacitated because of my strokes, they act as if I am already dead.

At first I believed it was my fault, but I don't think that's true. When I am with people, I don't bitch about being sick, and I try very hard to be interesting. No matter how I act, my old friends do not want to see me. I think people are afraid of illness and that's why they run away from those of us who are incapacitated.

I'm more lonely than you can imagine.

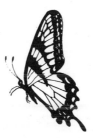

13

Tamara
Lupus Helped Me Grow

My psychotherapist asked me, "Is there anything positive that your lupus has done for you?"

I was startled and a little offended. She should have known better. I had been seeing her once a week for several months, and had spent the time telling her the negatives of my struggle with lupus. I shared my worries that I wouldn't be able to keep up with others at work and that my career would be blocked by lupus. I described my pain and my days of incapacity, exhaustion, and depression. I hadn't exaggerated. Lupus brings the worst pain imaginable, and total fatigue.

I described to her my difficulties with Patrick, my lover of more than seven years. I told her that since lupus he had changed from a romantic, wonderful lover into a perpetually angry and dissatisfied man. I blamed lupus for that, too. She should have known better than to insinuate that lupus had done anything positive for me.

I sat silently in her office, and then I heard myself say one faint word, "boundaries." I thought about the word and what it had come to mean for me. "Because of lupus, I am learning the importance of boundaries."

For the first year of our relationship, Patrick and I had a long-distance romance, because we lived 500 miles apart. We talked on the phone almost every evening, and got to know each other well by sharing our past experiences, attitudes, desires, and emotions. Every other weekend we were together. We made love, danced, listened to music, talked easily, and went on elaborate shopping trips for food. He was cook and I played the role of assistant cook, washing the food, chopping, and cleaning up, while he lingered over the bubbling pots, tasting and adding special seasonings.

Because we were newly in love, whatever we did seemed intimate and beautiful. I was an attractive size eight in those days; he, too, was trim, so we were a good-looking couple.

On the few occasions when I wasn't at home to receive his evening calls, he was upset, and wanted to know where I'd been, but that didn't bother me. I told myself his interrogations proved he loved me, and I think that was true. I learned very early in our relationship that he could be jealous and possessive, and needed to win arguments, but I didn't care. I wasn't perfect either and, besides, I believed that when he got to know and trust me more, he'd change.

I could see another problem, which I also ignored. He liked telling me what to do and how to do it, and I must have had inklings that someday I would resent this, even though at first it was lovely to have someone care enough about my life to want make decisions for me. Patrick said very candidly that I was more independent than other women he had dated, and that was tricky for him, although he admired the fact that I had a good job and did well at it. I can say honestly that Patrick was a very good man, who wanted to be appreciated, and I appreciated him. There were so many positives in our relationship that I was sure we would overcome our minor difficulties.

The twice-a-month weekends gave me something exciting to look forward to, without my having to be "up" all the time. To me, "up" meant being keenly aware of Patrick, in order to do what would be most pleasing to him. I wanted very much for him to be happy with me, and he was. We were a beautiful, competent couple, and in love.

After a year of long-distance dating, I applied for and got a nice promotion and job transfer to the city where Patrick lived. I was thrilled! We went house-hunting, and signed a lease to rent a small house together. I brought my things, he brought his, and we bought a few things together, to make our home new and special.

We had some minor difficulties. Patrick complained whenever I worked overtime, and he didn't like my new friends from my work. I alternated between arguing with him and reassuring him that he was the most important person in my life and that I loved him very much. I knew that in the past he had been hurt by other women, and I wanted to prove to him that I was not like them. I toned down my own desires and beliefs, while catering to his. I encouraged Patrick to continue his before-work breakfasts with a group of men who had been his friends since childhood. Perhaps that would help him realize that I, too, needed friends of my own.

All in all, we loved each very much and had hopes and plans for a long future together. Our love life was superb.

I passed my probationary period at work with flying colors, and received another raise in pay. My job was the best I could imagine, stimulating and creative, and I enjoyed the people I was working with. I told Patrick enthusiastically, "Everything's going my way!"

And then lupus struck suddenly and hard. The pain was terrible. I was hospitalized for a week, stayed at home another week, and afterwards it was all I could do to get to the office and survive through each day. I was terrified and depressed, because I was so very sick and the sickness was so crazy. One day I would believe I was dying, and a week later I would feel relatively well. I couldn't understand what was going on in my body, nor could I predict from one day to the next what my symptoms would be.

I was constantly worried that I might have to stop working. I suppose that is a worry facing all lupus patients who like or need their jobs. I had purchased disability insurance, but my self-esteem was involved. It was vitally important to me that I earn my own money and be independent. To be unemployable would be far more terrible than to be in pain. I love my work.

At first, Patrick was very supportive and caring. He asked a lot of questions about the disease, and he read the articles about lupus that my doctor loaned me. He came to the lupus support group and listened carefully to the other lupus patients. He learned to give me shoulder massages, but he refused to understand that sometimes a massage is wonderful and at other times it causes even more pain. I think he felt personally rejected whenever his efforts didn't bring me relief.

As before, I focused more on Patrick than on myself. Instead of doing what I could to take care of myself, I was expending energy taking care of Patrick's feelings. I would try to explain what was going on with me, but he didn't understand. I think he could have tolerated very well a brief, severe illness in which he could be a hero as he helped me through it. Lupus is a lifetime calamity, and that is much too long for many partners to endure.

As time when on, I felt less and less supported by him. One major problem was that his way of coping with an awful truth is to deny its existence. Therefore, he didn't admit to himself that I was very sick. For example, in the past I had worked overtime and he had taken this as a personal affront. Now, whenever I was a few minutes late, he'd accuse me of working overtime rather than coming home to him.

I tried to placate him. "I never work overtime any more. They don't even expect me to. I'm late because it takes awhile to get home."

"You weren't there when I called," he insisted loudly.

"I was at work all day. Where else would I be?" Inside, I was beginning to seethe. Where in hell did he think I was? Did he think I was carrying on a second romance, when I was too sick to do anything beyond surviving?

"I phoned your office and they said you'd left an hour ago."

"I was parked by the side of the freeway, sleeping. I was too tired to drive straight home. I can't help being so tired."

Some evenings I physically could not drive thirty minutes without a rest along the way. That may sound crazy to anyone who hasn't had lupus, but very often at the end of a difficult day, I had to pull off the freeway to take a nap.

Although angry, I would try hard to get him to understand. I thought that if I were patient and loving, he would begin to grasp what I was going through. As my disease continued, I told myself that I was lucky to have Patrick, because he was sticking by me in spite of lupus. I knew that men, especially when they weren't married, often desert a sick partner.

We had other disagreements. Many evenings I needed to go to bed as soon as I got home. My body demanded it. This was a real disappointment for Patrick, because dinner was important to him. After we both got home, he expected me to go grocery shopping with him and then help him cook, when all I wanted to do was lie down and rest.

I would give in and go to the store with him, but when we returned with the groceries, I'd be exhausted and in so much pain that I'd go right to bed. He'd be furious that he had to cook and eat alone, and would pay me back by leaving a mess in the kitchen for me to clean. Usually, I would not feel up to it, and that would start new arguments. We needed to hire a cleaning person, but didn't. Adding to all of my other worries, I was becoming afraid to spend money, because I didn't know when I might have to give up my job.

The days when I was comparatively well, I would cook with him and we'd go to a movie or watch a video together. That was fine. The trouble came when I wanted to go to a company party or to a friend's home. There were many business-related festivities: birthdays, wedding showers, picnics, and special parties whenever an important contract had been obtained or fulfilled, and I wanted to attend these whenever possible. "If you're well enough for your friends, why aren't you well enough for me?" he'd argue.

Over and over, I'd explain to Patrick that lupus was a crazy disease. I could be energetic one day and then sick for several days in a row. He refused to accept that I had enough energy for a party tonight, when just a few days before I had been too tired to go out with him. He believed that if my activities had to be restricted because of lupus, I should give up friends and save all my time for him.

The stress in our home was hurtful to me. I just had to get away from him sometimes, to be with my new women friends from work so that I could bitch about my life with lupus, without starting a fight. I found it easier to be with friends than with Patrick. With friends, I didn't have to defend myself or censor what I wanted to say. As I worked hard to be agreeable and keep Patrick happy, I became more and more depressed.

I was still convinced that if only I could help Patrick understand what was going on with me, he'd be accepting of the way I was running my life. Lupus is difficult for anyone to understand. Patrick didn't seem to believe that my whole body could be hurting horribly without showing any signs, such as bruises, swelling, or scars. There is no visible proof of illness, except for an occasional rash, which is really quite minor, and, of course, the nasty reality that steroids had ballooned me from a lovely size eight into a bloated size fourteen.

I guess it is understandable that a suspicious person would decide that I was faking, and that's exactly what Patrick decided. He said I got well whenever it was convenient for me. I almost wished that I needed braces, crutches, or any visible symptoms to prove that I was ill.

I adopted a "work till you drop" attitude, because I realized I was truly on my own. He was not good for me emotionally or financially. I seemed to be having increased difficulties with lupus. I had more flares and was using more steroids with fewer positive results. The pain in my joints was increasing.

I couldn't predict the future, but I did know in my heart that if my health deteriorated to the point where I needed a care-taker, Patrick would not be willing to take care of me.

I joined a lupus support group, which was a real break-through for me. I was so relieved to hear other women voice the same complaints I had, that friends and family don't be-lieve the extent of our illness.

I started to pay more attention to my body and to be aware of how I felt in different situations and with different people. I analyzed my daily activities as well as my emotions, and learned that some situations and some people's company recharged me, while others seemed to drain me.   Some people were natu-rally soothing or optimistic, and I found them easy to be with. Patrick was loud, argumentative, and draining. Our relation-ship was based too much on what we did for each other, and I felt guilty as I realized that he worked hard to make house re-pairs, help me in the garden, cook, and shop. He insisted that we spend almost all our time interacting, talking, making love, cooking together. For him even arguing was better than simply sitting in the same room, reading. He didn't like the quietness that I needed. Though he remained a wonderful lover, I wasn't well enough to endure these other facets of his personality that I used to find challenging and romantic.

I still told myself that all long-term relationships require work, and so I tried to explain gently to Patrick how I wanted us to relate. Unfortunately, he considered my views to be a put-down. He tried to be good to me, he said, and I agreed that this was true. I also agreed that he did a great deal for both of us.

I continued to believe that I was the one who had to do the changing of both him and me, to make him less angry and to make me more tolerant, and since I failed, I stayed depressed, guilty, anxious, and angry. These feelings were harmful, use-less, and were draining away my vitality. I had to begin to take better care of myself, physically and emotionally. As a first step, I found myself a psychotherapist. At first, I spent therapy hours weeping, which didn't accomplish much but was a relief.

Then, quite suddenly, I "got it." I stopped being guilty. I stopped defending myself against Patrick's jealousy, and refused to believe that I could hurt him. When he brought up a past hurt, I would respond, "We've already talked about that and I consider the issue resolved."

I explained that I enjoyed evenings with him, when I wasn't too sick to stay up, but I was not going to have unpleasant times. I would not revert to arguing, defending, or feeling guilty. It was hard to change my old ways of being, but I kept at it because I knew my health was at stake.

It was amazing how much better I began to feel as soon as I realized that I was in charge of my happiness and he was in charge of his!

I refused to let him put a damper on my happiness. It was hard enough being sick with lupus, without adding emotional misery to my physical pain.

I stopped trying to do more than felt right to me. I used part of my salary to hire a weekly cleaning woman. I told Patrick that, much as I loved his food, I was willing to pay for take-out food, and quiet.

Patrick didn't understand. He kept reminding me of everything he had done for me and all the sacrifices he had made for me (mostly imagined), and insisted that I do more for him. I had become selfish, he said. I ignored these invitations to battle.

Because I wouldn't argue any more, we didn't talk much. More and more, I spent evenings by myself, reading and resting, and felt a new internal peacefulness. I continued therapy, and kept learning more about my own boundaries. Finally, I knew that Patrick and I were not going to change enough to stay together.

By mutual consent we ended our seven-year relationship, which had begun with so much joy and hopefulness. I was sad about that, because a dream had ended. So was Patrick.

Although I missed Patrick, I found that my longings were for the way we had been at the beginning of our relationship, when I was healthy. From the beginning, I was a placater, as I let him intrude into my space. I hadn't understood that I needed to define my own boundaries, rather than permit him to define them for me. I will never again choose a lover who tells me what I ought to do, think, or feel.

I now say "No" without feeling selfish. I am alone, but not lonely. I eat and sleep when I choose. It is my responsibility to take care of myself. I have peace of mind. I respect myself, and that is incredibly important. Lupus provided the impetus for me to change, and my changes were at first painful but also life-affirming. Yes, there are positives that have come from my struggle with lupus.

After Patrick and I split up, I decided that lupus and romance just didn't go together for me. I saw no possibility that I would meet a man who would accept me the way I am now. But several months ago I began dating someone who works at my office. He's kind, generous, and the low-key type who likes to go out once in a while but is also content at home with me.

I am now healthier, I think, but the important part is that I am happy and therefore don't agitate myself about my health. Flares or not, I am happy at home and at work, and optimistic about my future. We're moving slowly in our relationship, and I do love him.

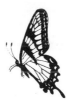

14

Gregory
Exercise Got Me Sailing Again

So, I'm the first male in your lupus book! Just ask me any thing you want to know. I'm divorced, no children, age forty-eight.

When did I find out I had lupus? You might say that I had a very crowded summer two years ago, with lupus and colon cancer. It all seemed to start after Memorial Day weekend. On Sunday I sailed on San Francisco Bay and after the race I bicycled through the Marin headlands, and then on Monday I bicycled Twin Peaks, which is a strenuous and wonderful ride. Afterwards I thought I must have overdone it, because I became so lethargic. The following Saturday all I could do was ride my bike through Golden Gate Park, and very slowly at that. Then things began to develop, and I couldn't bicycle again for over half a year.

What developed? Pains. They were very strange. Other people talk about pain in their joints, but what I had was pain in my muscles. Fortunately, I had insurance. I'm a writer by profession, and just a few months before this craziness in my muscles, I was between assignments. In fact, I'd gotten right to the edge of "How do I pay the next month's rent?" so I took a job with a computer company to tide me over, and that's why I have fine insurance. I don't know what I would have done if I'd been completely on my own.

I saw a doctor, who said that I was somewhat anemic, so he ordered a colonoscopy and found a small cancer in my colon. They didn't want to remove it until they knew what else was wrong, because cancer couldn't have been the cause of my muscle problems. They tested me for Lyme's Disease, AIDS, bacterial infection, everything they could think of, and they found I had lupus. The doctor told me the name, SLE, and what medicine he would prescribe, and said nothing else at all about the disease. No explanation and no practical information. He didn't even tell me to stay out of the sun.

When they took out the cancer, the strangest thing happened. Immediately after the surgery, I was fine! I had no pain in my muscles. In spite of my colon surgery, the first time I got out of bed, I stood on one leg and raised my other leg as high as I could, as if I were doing a place kick in football, and I shouted "Whoopee!" I thought I was well.

That didn't last long. When I got home from the hospital, not only did the pain recur, but the muscles stopped working. I couldn't pick up a glass or do the dishes. I stumbled and tripped over my own feet just walking across the living room floor. I couldn't even pull on my own underpants. I was recovering from the surgery and going through states of incontinence, wearing pads, and my hands were almost useless. With my incontinence and inability to walk, I couldn't leave my apartment.

Since I couldn't go to the library to look for a book on lupus, I phoned my brother, who found someone with the disease. She phoned and told me a lot about lupus and suggested I get in touch with the Lupus Foundation of America. I called them and asked how to sign up. They sent me good information and suggested I join a support group.

When I felt well enough to go outside, I could barely walk. If I came to the slightest incline in the sidewalk, it would feel like a mountain. I began to ask myself, "How much of this am I willing to take? At what point do I want to stop living?" For me, this was important to decide.

No, I was not depressed. You must think that a person has to be depressed to think about checking out. That's not depression. That's making an assessment. Maybe this is a difference between men and women. Maybe women are more emotional and less physical, so they don't care as much when they lose physical abilities. What do you think? I am not the type to be sad. I am angry at what I can't do, and my anger keeps me fighting to do more.

Anyway, I decided to do everything I could to recover, but if I couldn't recover enough to ride my bike and sail, I'd check out of this life.

When I got around to telling my friends what had been happening to me, they rallied for me. That was the only bright spot. I found out how many good friends I have! People dropped by to take me out for a bowl of soup or just to talk.

I took Prednisone for ten weeks, and then was put on Plaquenil. I designed my own exercise regime. I had never worked out in a gym before, but I decided that was a good first step. Even before I could hold a dish, I was using a weight machine. When I could hold things again, someone at the gym suggested I practice holding a hammer at arm's length and twisting my arm, so I forced myself to do it, and that helped, too. Another person recommended a physical rehabilitation center that specializes in hands, and those physical therapists did a lot for me. It took twenty weeks to get back on my bike. That's a hell of a long time for someone who's as impatient as I am.

People suggested acupuncture and massage, but I couldn't afford it, because my insurance didn't cover them. Others brought me herbs that I tried, but they didn't seem to do me any good, so I quit them. They say it takes months for herbs to work, and I don't have much faith in the idea of eating an herb in order to be stronger. I did change my diet. I got off my regular diet of hamburgers and coffee, and now I eat lots of fruits and vegetables.

I'm not well. The chest, for instance. Something is wrong in there. I can't sneeze. It's strange. I feel the urge, take a breath and can't sneeze. So I do breathing exercises and it is better than it was. I have pulmonary tests coming up.

I am fascinated by what this disease does to people. Each day or month is different. Just the other day I lost feeling in my toes. They were cold and numb. When a new symptom occurs, you wonder what else will happen to you? It's both fascination and dread. My brother's friend says her lupus is affecting her brain, and that's no good.

At work, I still find it difficult to keep up. After about five hours, I am tired. Maybe I'm really only a five-hour-a-day man. I do walk back and forth to work, to keep building myself up, but the walk home is tough. I bicycle every weekend, but I'm not ready for Twin Peaks yet. Mostly I take short trips on level ground. Of course, I have learned to wear the right clothes to guard against the sun.

The big gain for me is, I'm sailing again, even though it's incredibly difficult to move from one side of a boat to the other, while keeping your butt low. I practice squatting exercises at home to strengthen the right muscles. You have to be able to move your butt quickly in a race. I don't try to pretend anything. I say, "Gosh, it hurts being in this boat. I have lupus!" People are understanding.

I belong to a club that has a few dinghies that anyone can use, but mostly I crew in other people's boats. It's the most wonderful feeling, being out on the Bay. You can't beat it. A friend wants to sail the Greek islands, and he's invited me to go with him. I plan on going, if I can figure out how to afford it. I think I can.

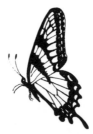

15

Tom
I Never Really Had A Life

Well, let's see. I'm thirty-six years old, I grew up in the rural south on a farm, and I got lupus when I was twelve years old. The things I've always hated most about lupus is tiredness, and the way I look. I have rashes on my face, between my fingers and in my hairline. I lose hair in clumps, it grows back, and I lose it again. Sometimes my eyebrows almost disappear. My face gets swollen and I have hyper-pigmentation on my face and neck. Sometimes I look very ugly, and sometimes I look more or less OK.

Off and on, I have pain in my hands, wrists, legs, and hips. I may look fine and feel terrible, or the other way around, so the way I look has nothing to do with the way I feel.

Lupus struck me without any warning. We had a large yard, about an acre, and one of my jobs was to take out the garbage. All of a sudden, I got so tired I'd even have to rest on my way back from taking out the garbage. How do you explain to anyone that you can't take out the garbage without resting?

My parents brought me to a doctor, who told my mother, "There is nothing wrong with that boy." So I had to shut up about how I felt.

In high school, I wrestled and played football, but I was always very tired. I'd go to bed before 8 pm every night, and I had no energy for school work or a social life. I was in sports to prove I could do it, but I never liked them because I felt so sick.

After I graduated from high school, I began to have a lot of problems that seemed to come out of nowhere, like severe ear infections. I got very sick from the sun. I swelled up, was nauseated, and my knees and hips hurt so much that I couldn't bear to straighten my legs. I wished I could scream, I hurt so much. My face swelled up, and I couldn't recognize myself when I looked in the mirror.

I kept asking myself why I was sick, and I decided it was just my fate. I never understood why all these things happened to me. I never smoked or drank or used drugs. I didn't go to parties. I ate well and never let myself get fat. I would wonder if I was a little bit crazy, but then I'd say to myself, "No, I'm not crazy. I'm not imagining all this."

I began seeing a variety of doctors, and I was always apologetic to them. I felt ashamed to take up their time, since none of them seemed to believe I really was sick. Finally, when I was twenty-five, I went into the hospital because of the pain in my legs and hips. This time I saw a woman doctor, who X-rayed my joints and told me there was nothing wrong with them, but she didn't just dismiss me the way other doctors did. She took me at my word. She said, "I don't know what is wrong with you, but I am going to find out." That was the first time a doctor said anything like that to me.

She sent me to a big research hospital in our state. When I got there, an intern asked what was wrong, and I told him every symptom I had since I was twelve. It took a long time. I saw dozens of interns, and talked about my symptoms for hours. One of them asked if I could have picked up a fungus or something in Vietnam. I said, "Not hardly, since I have never been there, and I've never even known anyone who went."

Finally, a doctor said, "I really don't want to tell you this because you're a male and so young, but you have lupus." He said, "It's chronic. You'll never be rid of it," and he reeled off the names of the medication he was going to prescribe.

I said, "No!" I stood up and left, and never went back. You see, I felt hopeless. After all these years, I found out I would never be well. My self-esteem was destroyed. I kept thinking,

"Who would want to be around a person like me? Who'd want to know a person who has to go to bed at 8:00 every night and can't go anywhere, who has rashes and is ugly? Who'd want to know anybody whose sickness was chronic?" I was devastated. The worst part was the feeling that I didn't have control over my body. I couldn't make it do what I wanted it to do, and it would be that way for the rest of my life.

Finally, I decided to move across the country and start over. That was a giant step for someone like me. For the past 8 years, I've worked for a small company here, building kitchen cabinets. I live alone with my dog and my books. I read all the time. Up to now, reading has been my life.

I went to one meeting of a lupus support group, but most of the members are women my mother's age, so I didn't go back. Recently I got a book on chess from the library and found out I like chess. I've joined a chess club. I'm only a beginner but the other players say I have a talent for it.

I'm going to a rheumatologist now, and taking Plaquenil. It's too early to say whether it's doing me any good. I've never really had a life, so I'm afraid to hope, if you know what I mean, but maybe my life is getting better.

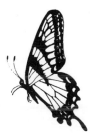

16

Vicky
My Nightmare With Drugs

I have what is called a mild case of lupus, which means lots of pain and exhaustion, but no life-threatening lupus in my vital organs. I've been taking Paxil, Plaquenil, and Feldene or Naprosyn for years.

When I experienced a new, severe flare of joint and muscle pain plus fatigue, my doctor prescribed 20 mg of Prednisone plus an antibiotic for swollen lymph glands. Three days later I ran out of Paxil, and the pharmacist refused to renew my prescription because his computer said it was "too soon." He said to come back in a week. (I found out later that the previous prescription was only partially filled, because he had run out of Paxil, and my remaining medication, with my name on it, had been on the pharmacist's shelf for weeks.)

I felt fine at first, without the Paxil. Because of having started Prednisone, I felt energetic, clear-minded, and happy. I decided that I could manage for a week without an anti-depressant. Two days later, I worked at my job all day and then spent the evening gardening. I didn't need or want sleep, and joked about installing flood lights in the garden so I could work all night. The next day I continued to work well on the job, and was happy about being able to accomplish so much. I was still energetic and happy that evening. Waking before dawn, I steam-cleaned all the rugs in the house, mopped the floors, and went to my job.

Toward evening, my excitement changed to agitation. I couldn't relax, and felt as if my internal gas pedal was stuck on "full speed ahead." I lay awake, and suddenly began to imagine that there had been a terrible highway accident and my son was killed. I even phoned hospitals to check, and was very upset until he came home. I have never before been worried about him in this way. When I finally fell asleep, I began having the most terrible nightmares of my life.

The next day at work I had a very tense quarrel with my boss, and had urges to attack her physically, although I am normally a very peaceful person. I kept my self-control and chose my words very carefully. Later, she told me she had been afraid of me because I seemed strange.

The next night, the nightmares began again, and I woke up terrified, mistaking shadows for strange people in my room. When I tried to scream I felt paralyzed. I was losing track of what was dream and what was reality.

The next morning, Sunday, I was dizzy, unable to stand alone, and I wouldn't close my eyes for fear of seeing the nightmares. I stopped all of my medications, including Prednisone, because I didn't know which of them might be responsible for my symptoms. I had to wait in this condition until my physician was available on Monday.

On Monday, when I saw the doctor, I was still very dizzy and couldn't walk alone. He put me back on Paxil, and attributed my mental symptoms to stopping an anti-depressant abruptly rather than gradually. We both decided against my going back on Prednisone because I was no longer suffering from the joint pain that initially warranted Prednisone. In two days the joint pain had returned, but I decided to use my non-steroidal anti-inflammatories for my pain, instead of Prednisone. Now I am fully recovered.

I had read about psychosis with lupus, but I never believed it could happen to me. I was so naive and prejudiced that I thought psychosis only occurred in people who were already on-the-edge, what you call "flakey." I am a normal woman who holds down a good job in spite of lupus, and although I have been taking the anti-depressant, I am not at all concerned about my mental health. Now I am concerned about medications!

In the future I will be much more cautious with medications, and will take the very least I can. I am gradually weaning myself from Paxil.

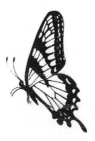

17

Medications

It's a relief to a lupus sufferer to get a diagnosis. After all the medical appointments, laboratory tests, and sometimes hospitalizations, you are probably glad to have a label that tells you what is wrong. You hope for and expect rapid, effective treatment plus relief from pain. Unfortunately, with lupus the relief you obtain may be incomplete and disappointing, and medications may bring a host of unpleasant and even dangerous side effects.

It is important for you to learn about the medications commonly prescribed for lupus. You'll want to understand both their benefits and their adverse side-effects, so that you can talk intelligently with your doctor about your treatment and let her know what is and is not working well for you. Here is a brief description of medications you may be given:

Nonsteroidal anti-inflammatory drugs (NSAID). For joint pain you may be treated initially with a mild NSAID. Your physician may suggest Lodine, Disalcid, Trilisate, or something similar. These are well tolerated by most people, and rarely upset the stomach. However, because these medications are mild, they are only effective with mild pain.

If the mild NSAIDs are not effective in reducing pain to a tolerable level, your physician may prescribe a stronger NSAID, such as Naprosyn, Feldene, or Indocin.

There are NSAIDs available without prescription that contain ibuprofen, which people take for occasional pain. They are not recommended for long-term use, because of the danger of ulcers or liver damage.

NSAIDs have both pain-relieving and anti-inflammatory benefits, but do not control or slow down the progression of the disease itself. They need to be taken every day to maintain a therapeutic blood level for their anti-inflammatory benefits, and should be taken with food to prevent stomach ulcers.

The most common adverse reactions to NSAIDs are a tendency to bleed easily, especially in the gastro-intestinal tract. You may notice a tendency to bruise easily. If you feel pain or a burning sensation in your abdomen or if your stools are black and tarry, let your doctor know immediately. She will order laboratory tests to determine if you have gastro-intestinal bleeding.

Another possible side effect is kidney damage. Kidney function needs to be monitored through lab tests. People with kidney problems, cannot take NSAIDs.

On rare occasions, a patient is allergic to NSAIDs, and may develop asthma, which clears up when the medication is discontinued.

NSAIDs are not compatible with some over-the-counter medications, so it is important for your physician to know everything you are taking, including non-prescription drugs.

Narcotics. For acute episodes of severe pain, narcotics, such as Vicodin and morphine, are prescribed. They are limited to short-term use, because of their addictive potential and negative impact on the patient's ability to maintain such normal daily activities as working and driving.

Anti-malarials. Anti-malarial medication, most commonly Plaquenil, may be prescribed for skin rashes and joint pain, and to slow the progress of the disease. (Discoid lupus skin lesions that do not respond to topical creams will respond to anti-malarials.) The use of anti-malarials was discovered by accident, when soldiers, who were given anti-malarial drugs prior to going to countries where there was malaria, felt much less joint pain.

Anti-malarials are relatively mild and safe for long-term use, suppress flares, and help reduce inflammation. The benefits to your joints will not be felt immediately, so don't give up if at first it doesn't seem to help. You will be taking this medication over a long period of time. It can be taken safely with Prednisone and anti-inflammatories, including aspirin.

The only known side effect, which is extremely rare, is retinal damage. Therefore, anyone taking Plaquenil, should be examined by an ophthalmologist (eye doctor.)

Steroids, most commonly Prednisone, are used for severe pain that is not relieved by the non-steroidal medications, and for lupus disease affecting kidneys, heart, lungs, or central nervous system. Steroids treat symptoms, pain and inflammation, and suppress the disease itself. In SLE myositis, which causes weakness, pain, and deterioration in muscles, steroids must be given in high dosages initially for prompt suppression and control of the myositis. With myositis, the client also needs physical therapy with a good exercise program to regain normal muscle strength and function. This is what Gregory designed for himself so that he could bicycle and sail again.

Prednisone is similar to corticosteroids produced by your adrenal glands. While you are taking Prednisone, your adrenal glands' production of this steroid is temporarily suppressed. That is why an abrupt discontinuation of Prednisone can cause serious, even life-threatening, withdrawal symptoms as well as a severe flare of your lupus.

Prednisone can cause insomnia, so should be taken in the morning. There are other major side effects, including: facial rash or acne; fat deposits in the abdomen, hips, back of the neck, and face; facial hair; mood alterations such as depression or irritability; muscle weakness or atrophy in legs and arms; thinning of the skin and easy bruising; loss of calcium in the bones, which can result in osteoporosis and subsequent fractures; increase in blood sugar, leading to diabetes; increased risk of infection; cataracts; and temporary psychosis.

In spite of these side effects, you may need to take steroids. They may save your life. The side effects are more likely to occur when steroids are taken for a long period of time. They should be used during flares and medical crises, and then discontinued as soon as possible.

Chemotherapeutic drugs, such as Cytoxin or Imuran, are prescribed when there is serious organ involvement, such as severe kidney disease. Methotrexate, another chemotherapeutic drug, is used for incapacitating joint pain. These medications are used when a person cannot take NSAID or steroids. They have serious side effects, including damage to blood cells and increased susceptibility to infections and cancer.

Etidronate, or Didronel is used in the prevention and treatment of osteoporosis, a crippling bone disease. In the past it was prescribed to fortify brittle bones in the elderly, and recently has been found to be beneficial in treating lupus patients who take steroids.

Many lupus patients have other autoimmune diseases, such as Hashimoto's Thyroiditis, Sjogrens syndrome, colitis, or rheumatoid arthritis. They need additional medications if they have more than one autoimmune disorder. For example, Hashimoto's thyroiditis is an autoimmune disease which attacks the thyroid, so thyroid replacement pills are prescribed.

Lupus patients may have medical problems unrelated to lupus, such as high blood pressure, gastro-intestinal problems, or seizure disorders, which require additional medications. Some of these medications interact unfavorably with lupus medications and may affect the patient's sense of well-being. For example, Dilantin, used for control of seizures, will increase fatigue in the lupus patient. Again, it is vital that you and your doctor know what you are taking, and that you don't add new medications or discontinue old ones without your doctor's approval.

Anti-depressants. Depression often accompanies lupus. It may be caused by the lupus itself, or by the medications prescribed to treat lupus; or it may be the emotional reaction to having this painful, unpredictable, chronic disease. When depressed, patients may experience inertia, lethargy, irritation or agitation, sudden bouts of tears, suicidal thoughts, and feelings of hopelessness and helplessness.

Physicians commonly prescribe antidepressants, such as Prozac, Zoloft, Wellbutrin, or Paxil. In addition to their antidepressant effects, these medications may increase a person's level of energy, and alleviate fatigue.

Side effects with antidepressants include: blurred vision, tremors, agitation, tingling in hands and feet, decreased sex drive, palpitations, tightness in the throat, dry mouth, constipation or diarrhea, sweating, rashes, insatiable appetite that leads to excessive weight gain, and may occasionally cause increased depression. If you experience any of these side effects, inform your physician. You may want to reduce or discontinue the medications, but you must do this gradually. Vicki (Chapter 16) tells her harrowing experience with suddenly stopping her antidepressant drug.

The research and marketing of new medication is ongoing, so patients may receive prescriptions with unfamiliar names. Ask your doctor about any new medication and be aware of possible side-effects.

Remember to keep a list of all medications you are taking, plus any new or unusual sensations or symptoms that may be caused by them. Don't stop taking your medication if you don't like the way you feel. Instead, phone your pharmacist or physician. Pharmacists are great resources, because their specialty is medication and they get lots of feedback from their customers. Anyone with a chronic disease needs to make friends with her pharmacist. Find one who will take the time to talk with you about your medications.

18

Complementary Treatments

There are many beneficial treatments in addition to those your physician recommends. Sometimes they are called new-age or alternative treatments, but a better name is complementary treatments, because they are not substitutes for the medications you are taking.

Some treatments are new. Others, such as acupuncture, yoga, and herbal medicine have been around for thousands of years. In recent times, herbs are being tested in many parts of the world. Some are used extensively in Asia or Europe, but have not yet been tested in the United States.Medical students are seldom taught about complementary medicine, since the focus of their training is fighting disease rather than preventing it. The medical field today is beginning to focus somewhat more on prevention, as well as alternative methods to make people healthier. Howard Press (chapter 21) suggests that disease is basically a set of cells in a person's body that are not working properly, and that a fundamental priority must be to look for nutrients that can make new, better, healthier cells. Every nutritional advantage is important when the immune system is malfunctioning.

There are disadvantages to some of the new age treatments. Reliable information about them may be difficult to obtain, the products themselves may be untested, and for you they may be expensive simply because health plans probably won't reimburse you for their cost. If you choose to experiment, discuss with your physician what new treatments you are trying. You may find that she is glad to learn about complementary methods and will be interested in whether they work for you.

Practitioners. Non-medical practitioners include nutritionists, chiropractors, acupuncturists, homeopaths, kinesiologists, physical therapists, massage practitioners, and others. They have a bewildering assortment of skills, training, and approaches. To choose one of these practitioners, seek referrals from your friends and members of your lupus support group, and get a listing of approved providers from your health plan. Health book stores, independent book stores, and libraries have lots of books on alternative practitioners. A good description of many of these disciplines can be found on the internet: **http://www.altmedicine.com**

Nutrition. It would be nice if your food gave you all the nutrients that you need. Sufficient vitamins should be obtainable in the food we eat, but most of the time fruits and vegetables are vitamin-deficient, because the food was grown in depleted soil or was picked before it was ripe. To eat well you need vitamin and mineral supplements.

Eat low-fat protein, such as fish and white meat of poultry. If you are a vegetarian, you already know about tofu, powdered vegetable protein, and veggie burgers, but anyone can profit from adding these to her diet.

Limit your intake of fat, especially fatty meats, and hydrogenated oils such as margarine, mayonnaise, and butter. They add pounds you don't need, plus fatty acids that aggravate swelling and pain. Use olive oil and other vegetable oils instead.

Vegetables lead the list of foods that are good for you, packing a big load of vitamins and minerals per calorie. Let your carbohydrates come from fruits and vegetables, and go easy on bread, pasta, and desserts. Whole fruits and vegetables are far better than juice, because juice has an excess of sugar and no fiber. Because your vegetables may be vitamin-deficient, take supplements.

The vitamin A you need is found in yellow and green vegetables and fruit: apricots, carrots, sweet potatoes, broccoli and spinach.

Vitamin C is in most fresh fruits, sprouts, asparagus, and red peppers. Because vitamin C is destroyed easily by heat, it is best to cook vegetables very lightly, or serve them raw in salads.

Vitamin D is in milk, fish oils, and sunshine. Since you can't be in the sun, drink milk, and/or take supplementary vitamin D.

Flaxseed oil and cold water fish oils (Omega 3, not Omega 6) are said to aid your body in creating its own substance that relieves inflammation. Some people also consider these oils helpful in reducing the number of flares they experience.

Vitamin E is found in many foods, including vegetable oils, wheat germ, nuts, spinach, broccoli, and dried prunes.

You need calcium for maintaining strong bones. Anyone taking Prednisone must take extra calcium daily to counter-act the negative effect that Prednisone has on your bones.

Talk with a new-age nutrition counselor. Get books on nutrition from your health food bookstore, health store, independent bookstore, or public library. Use your computer (see Appendix) to keep abreast of the newest ideas about vitamins and other food supplements. That way, you can make your own educated choices about the food you eat.

There are almost as many ideas about diet and diet supplements as there are patients with lupus. Herbs and other nutritional supplements are usually more gentle than drugs, so you may have to take them for a period of time before seeing results. There are almost no negative side effects.

One type of nutritional supplement that has recently been widely recommended is anti-oxidants, which include vitamins C and E, and selenium. These are found naturally in sun-ripened fruit, but if the fruit is picked before it is ripe, it cannot manufacture its own anti-oxidants.

Grape seed extract seems to be an especially valuable anti-oxidant for lupus patients. Users claim that it counteracts inflammation, decreases allergic reaction, and repairs damaged collagen (connective tissue.)

Some people get immediate results. Some take anti-oxidants for weeks before they experience improvement. One woman with joint pain did not notice a benefit from grape seed extract until after four months of continued use, but since then has had very little pain. Grape seed extract or other anti-oxidants must be taken on a regular basis, not just when joints hurt.

Lupus patients might want to test a product called Juice-Plus, which has received rave notices on the internet. It is in capsule form and supplies needed anti-oxidants as well as fiber, trace minerals, and trace enzymes. It is made from fruit and vegetable concentrates plus added vitamins. The natural sugar has been removed, so diabetics can use it without problems. Your health food store has several similar products which are cheaper, such as Nature's Plus Ultra Juice and Nature's Life Greens.

Warning when shopping for food supplements: Avoid anything designed to stimulate your immune system, because yours is already over-stimulated. Echinacea, often combined with Goldenseal, has become very popular to ward off colds, and reduce their severity. It fights infection by stimulating the immune system, so it is **not** recommended for people with lupus. Another no-no is anything that contains alfalfa, because it aggravates lupus symptoms.

New Age Medicines. You can learn of new products on the internet, as well as in health magazines that emphasize holistic and natural medicines. Here are some ideas that may be helpful to you:

DHEA (dehydroespiandrosterone) is a naturally-occurring hormone precursor that has been widely advertised. Studies have shown that DHEA makes it possible to decrease dosages of steroids, and the side effects are milder. Physicians can't prescribe DHEA except for research studies, since it has not yet been approved by the FDA (Federal Drug Administration,) but it is available in health food stores. Because it is in the process of being tested, long term effects are not yet known.

Glucosamine and Chondroitin are two natural substances that are now considered very good alternatives to drugs in the treatment of osteoarthritis, which is caused in many lupus patients by the steroids they need to take.

Veterinarians first used these substances with arthritic animals, and then physicians in Europe began testing their effectiveness with humans. Lupus patients are now using Glucosamine and Chondroitin in the United States, as well as in Europe, with good results. Patients report lessened pain, reduced swelling, and healing of joints. Glucosamine and Chondroitin are non-toxic and have no known side effects even with prolonged use.

Are you a person who likes Tiger Balm, that strong salve that has been used for centuries to ease pain? If you are, there is something new for you, not nearly so hot, called Arth-Rx, a non-prescription remedy sold in pharmacies. It's a liquid that rolls onto the skin, like a roll-on deodorant. It warms the skin and seems effective in reducing pain.

Marijuana is beneficial in suppressing pain and nausea. It is deeply relaxing and brings a sense of well-being to people who are suffering. It is to be hoped that medical indications for its use will be specified and approved, so that its benefits can be available to those who need it.

There are many herbal medicines, with ingredients that only herbal specialists recognize. That is the problem. Because the names of the herbs are unfamiliar, it's difficult to know what you are taking and whether there are side effects. Probably your best bet, if you want to try herbal medicine, is to obtain it from someone who has studied Eastern medicine and can explain the ingredients. A disclaimer: It is impossible to tell with any certainty what causes a person suddenly to feel better. When this occurs, a patient tends to give credit to whatever she was using at the time. When someone tells you of a miracle treatment, research it before committing yourself to its use.

Exercise. Exercise is a painful subject for people with lupus. Though it should be part of everyone's health regimen, many people with lupus avoid exercise, either because it hurts too much or they feel too tired to undertake it. Next time you wake up stiff and exhausted, try an experiment. Do some mild exercises. You may be amazed to discover that exercise, when done gently, decreases your exhaustion, and doesn't add to your pain.

Exercise is vital to optimum health. Gregory (Chapter 14) dedicated himself to finding the right exercises for regaining his lost physical abilities. He had severe pain in his muscles, could barely walk, and couldn't hold anything in his hands. He designed his own exercise program, working out in a gym, exercising at home, and getting physical therapy. He said, "It took twenty weeks before I had recovered enough to get back on my own bicycle." To him it was worth the struggle.

Osteoporosis, one of the debilitating conditions of aging, is especially common in lupus patients. You will be taking calcium, of course, to prevent osteoporosis, but tests have proven that weight-bearing exercises, such as walking and climbing stairs, outshine pills in keeping your bones strong. Bicycling puts less strain on your joints, but it is a limited-weight-bearing exercise, so isn't as effective for increasing bone mass.

Aerobic exercises increase your breathing capacity and endurance, and strengthen your heart. Good aerobic exercises include walking quickly, climbing stairs, dancing, bicycling, and swimming. Swimming, although not a weight-bearing exercise, is a fine aerobic exercise for people with tender joints.

You can swim laps, tread water, or join an aerobic exercise class at your local pool.

Physical therapists and trainers who have experience with lupus patients are wonderfully useful in helping you find the right exercises to strengthen your body. Find out if your insurance will pay for their help when your doctor signs a recommendation for it.

Yoga is a healing system for your body, mind, and spirit. Benefits from yoga include: increased flexibility and strength in your body, decreased stiffness and soreness, improvement in your circulation, stimulation of abdominal organs that results in better digestion, and restored spinal alignment. As Beth (chapter 11) reported, "When I can't get to sleep because my joints hurt, I get out of bed and do yoga stretching positions. It takes away the pain. I go to sleep more quickly and sleep more soundly."

You will want a good teacher, who understands your limitations and works well with you. Look for a group that welcomes older people as well as those with disabilities. It's more fun when you learn to do yoga with people at your own level. As you progress in yoga, you'll notice that you become more and more peaceful. Yoga is good for the spirit as well as the body.

Tai chi is a highly refined yet very simple system of exercise that has been used in China for hundreds of years. It consists of relaxed breathing and slow, continuous, easy movements designed to refresh and develop the whole body. The interplay of stillness and slow movement is calming and a very fine antidote to stress. It develops elasticity and strength in your joints. Tai chi can be learned from a book on the subject, but it is, of course, much better to join a tai chi class. One of the real attractions is that no matter what your age or physical condition, you can do tai chi.

Supplementary Treatments. Acupuncture is an excellent treatment for chronic pain, and has other benefits as well. There are Asian acupunturists who learned their specialty before coming to the United States. They also "take pulses" to learn about the strength or weakness or imbalance of an organ and body systems. Some modern physicians, like Dr. Press, are studying and practicing this ancient Eastern treatment, in which very fine needles are placed in specific points of the body. Some practitioners use acupressure, without needles, or a mild electric stimulation. Many lupus sufferers report that they have been helped greatly by Eastern medical approaches.

Unfortunately, since most medical research in this country is funded by large drug companies, funds are not made available for the proper testing of acupuncture. The treatment will be expensive for you if your insurance company refuses to pay for it.

Massage is useful for stimulating circulation, and reducing anxiety, depression, and pain. Many people are touch-starved, so the experience of relaxing and being touched is intensely beneficial. There are many different forms of massage. You will want to find the type you like and, of course, a practitioner you both like and trust.

Some massage therapists use acupuncture principles, with pressure on "sore spots." As with all other aspects of your own life, you are in charge. During a massage, ask for more or less pressure, and tell the massage person which areas of your body are sore and which need extra attention.

Biofeedback training teaches you how to relax many so-called "involuntary" muscles, and is useful in pain reduction, rehabilitation of muscles, and lowering of blood pressure.

There are so many complementary treatments being offered these day that a patient could spend considerable time searching the Internet for new ideas, talking with nutritionists, and enjoying being a part of the world of New Age medicine.

19

Pregnancy and Lupus

Whether or not to have a child is a difficult decision for women with lupus. Twenty years ago, medical textbooks stated that women with SLE should not get pregnant, because of health risks to both mother and child. Research has led to increased understanding of the factors associated with lupus-related miscarriages, and can identify the autoantibody (antiphospholipid antibody) that is responsible for the majority of miscarriages with lupus.

Women who are at risk of giving birth to babies with neonatal lupus can be identified, and steps taken to treat heart block if it occurs. However, while you are pregnant, you won't be able to take many of the medications listed in chapter 17, because of the danger to the fetus. If you have kidney or heart disease, pregnancy is very dangerous to mother and fetus. Discuss the risks with your doctor before allowing yourself to become pregnant. If you are incapable of being pregnant, sometimes adoption is an alternative.

In addition to the medical aspects of pregnancy, you need to consider whether you are able to cope with and care for a child. Giving birth to or adopting a child is the most irrevocable decision you will ever make. People choose careers, change their minds, and find new careers. They marry and then may divorce. Children, on the other hand, are their parents' responsibility from the day they are born until they are at least eighteen. Some hang around the family home longer. You can't divorce them, exchange them for a different model, or throw them out, even though at times you may wish they'd hurry up and get old enough to leave home. Children are a major part of a mother's life, a burden or her greatest joy. Most likely, the child is both.

Child care may be more than you can handle physically, emotionally, or financially. Unlike your healthy friends, you can't raise a child alone. Do you have a capable partner who will be willing to be responsible for infant and child care, when you are tired or incapacitated? Have you financial support, so that you can hire child care if you need it?

Lots of partners are heroes during the "short haul," as Tamara (chapter 13) learned. Lupus is a "long haul" disease. What is your guess about your partner's long-term ability to care for a child? What is the evidence for your guess? Are there relatives who will help care for your child? How faithful will your partner and your relatives be in keeping their promises?

The decision to become pregnant is ultimately yours. You must listen to your doctor, and may choose to listen to friends, relatives, financial advisers, therapists, and especially to your partner. You alone will decide if you will accept the risks of pregnancy and the difficulties of caring for an infant and child. No one but you can make that decision, although a husband or partner needs to agree with your decision. Have your partner go with you to talk with a physician and perhaps a psycho-therapist if the two of you don't agree.

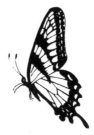

20

A Rheumatologist's Perspective
Interview: Joan Barber, M.D.

Patients come to me with complaints of joint pain, fatigue, and skin rashes, or are referred by family physicians because of similar complaints, the presence of a positive ANA test, or other symptoms or test results that suggest a connective tissue disease. About thirty percent of these patients have rheumatoid arthritis; fifty percent are classified as having an undifferentiated connective tissue disease, because their cases don't meet all of the criteria necessary for a diagnosis of a specific autoimmune disease; a few have one of the less common autoimmune diseases, such as Hashimoto's thyroiditis, scleroderma, polymyositis, Wegners vasculitis, Sjogrens syndrome, or drug-induced lupus; and about twenty percent have lupus.

The diagnosis of lupus is becoming increasingly more sophisticated, as we have available more refined blood tests.

At the first consultation, I spend at least an hour taking a thorough history, doing a physical exam, and ordering laboratory work. I ask the patient, "How are your symptoms affecting your life and your work?" "What do they prevent you from doing?" Using the patient's perspective as well as the results of lab tests, I determine how severe the disease is and how constant, frequent, or disabling the joint pain is. I prefer to give optimistic and encouraging information. I am extremely cautious about prematurely diagnosing lupus, until I am sure the label is correct. When I am sure, I remind the patient that ninety percent of lupus patients do not have organ involvement or a life-threatening disease. I don't want to instill unnecessary fear in a patient. I tell them lupus is a disease that can be identified, understood, and possibly controlled; and the progression of the disease can be slowed down.

I encourage patients to learn as much as possible about their disease. I am not enthusiastic about alternative therapy, because some health food preparations may be expensive and have hidden, dangerous side effects, and they are not well regulated. However, I would not criticize a patient for trying alternative treatments that are not dangerous, if that is something the patient wants to do for herself. It may have important psychological benefits.

I start my patients off with Plaquenil, which I consider to be safe and effective. Within a few months, the arthritis and rash will be reduced and flares will be less severe.

I want to see my patients every two - six months. During each visit I order blood tests and urinalysis to rule out lupus nephritis and other serious manifestations of lupus. I also do a physical exam, including looking for joint swelling, pleurisy, and changes in the skin. I ask patients about any new symptoms they may be experiencing, and check their medications.

Each time I see a patient, I want the patient to begin by describing any problems she may be having. How is the lupus affecting her life, work, and relationships? For example, "I can't change my baby's diapers because my hands are so stiff and sore," is important information I want to know immediately, not as the patient walks out the door. I don't want patients to hide their problems, even if the problems seem to them to be silly, unimportant, or frightening.

Sometimes even very intelligent people hide their real symptoms, because they are afraid of what the symptoms may reveal. They behave as if they believe that a serious problem will go away if it isn't talked about. The patient and I must discuss all concerns and problems, in order to find the best possible treatment for the unique aspects of each person's disease.

Relieving symptoms is not the same as treating the disease. Pain medication may mask the silent development of destructive arthritis or nephritis. For example, last week I saw a patient who had been put on a low-dose of Prednisone by a physician who kept refilling the prescription without seeing the patient. The patient believed she was doing well because Prednisone masked her discomfort. When I saw her, I discovered that she didn't have lupus at all. She had rheumatoid arthritis, which had gone untreated. Her hands showed on Xray deep erosions and bone destruction that could have been prevented. Merely feeling better should not make a patient over-confident.

Treatment needs to fit the level of the disease, balancing the risks of untreated lupus against the risks of the medication, be it Plaquenil, Prednisone, Imuran, or any prescribed medication.

Patients get the most out of their interactions with rheumatologists when they are willing to keep regular appointments, and work in partnership with the physician, sharing responsibilities and uncertainties.

I want to emphasize what a person can do, rather than catastrophize and dwell on what a person can't do. My desire for all patients is also their desire for themselves, the best possible quality of life. I encourage patients to continue with whatever makes their lives worthwhile, not to withdraw from life, and to keep moving beyond the limitations their disease may seem to impose. People can survive rough times and still be happy, productive, contributing, worth-while individuals.

Dr. Barber is a rheumatologist in Santa Cruz, California, who has been treating lupus patients for more than twenty years.

21

Self-Love, Self-Respect, and Self-Education
Interview: Howard Press, M.D.

When we talk about lupus, we need to start with the immune system. It is a system of defense that attacks noxious, foreign substances in the body. One of its functions is to distinguish the self from the non-self. Whenever the immune system, like any system, is overburdened and starts to fail, it begins to behave in an erratic manner. In lupus the over-burdened immune system begins to make antibodies against the body's own cells, as if the cells were foreign.

How does it become overburdened? The immune system is bombarded by a tremendous number of foreign antigens, micro-organisms, and parasites that enter our bodies and get into our bloodstream. This puts an ever-increasing strain on the immune system. The intact intestine acts as a selective barrier against this foreign matter, but if its membranes are inflamed and irritated, it won't be as effective, and that may increase the stress on the immune system.

Why do some immune systems break down when others do not? Perhaps some people are exposed to more toxic substances. And perhaps some are more fragile than others. People whose immune system is not working properly are among those who let the world know when all is not well in our environment, just as canaries let miners know when the air in coal mines becomes toxic. For these people, the toxic qualities of the world are more stressful, and their bodies go into an alarm state more readily.

Under environmental and internal pressure, the delicate, challenged immune system in some people breaks down and behaves in an aberrant fashion. One aberration is lupus.

Modern medicine makes war on disease, seeking to obliterate or suppress it. We attempt to eliminate whatever is harmful to the body, and what we can't eliminate, we attempt to suppress. There is nothing wrong with that. There's a place for suppressants, such as analgesics and steroids. If you are in terrible pain, your pain must be suppressed.

In medicine, we use the tools we have. We can't use the tools we don't know about or don't have, but we must remember that there is a much bigger set of tools out there. We need to seek out people who have other tools. I use tools from many sources. In addition to the tools I learned in medical school, I use acupuncture, herbal remedies, nutrition, exercise, anything that can enhance the patient's life.

We have to know where to look for new tools, and we have to be educated so that we make good choices. Discrimination is the key. Not everything advertised to be the latest, most wonderful cure turns out to be curative.

We also have to be optimistic and open. If we are not open, we don't look. What is not sought is never found. Every cure is somewhere in the universe, and we simply have to find it.

The body responds to physical, chemical, and biological laws of nature, just as a plant does. If you put a camellia in the sunlight, it's going to burn. Some plants grow in shade, some in sun, some in acid soil. Any two roses need different care, just like people. A healthy plant may have worms nearby that drain the nutrients and keep the plant from getting what it needs. Aphids may attack it. Weather conditions may be poor. To keep plants healthy, someone needs to care for them, put nutrients in the soil, spray, and water. Even if a plant is genetically strained, vulnerable, with inherent weakness, you can still do a lot to help it grow. A plant with a chronic disease, given good care, will do better than a healthy plant that is ignored. And so it is with people.

From my perspective, good health care includes both the person and the environment in which the person lives.

One of the problems of medical practice today is that we do not recognize the innate spiritual needs of human beings. When a sick or aged person is in an environment that is non-supportive, non-nutritive, that person closes down. In a nutritive environment that supports spiritual needs, she can go on and on.

Self-care is vital. What does self-care mean? It means that the individual is responsive and responsible rather than passive in the treatment of her illness. This requires self-love, self-respect, and self-education.

A passive person says to her doctor, "I don't want to make trouble," "I don't want to bother you," "I'm sorry I took your time," or "I don't have any questions." When the doctor gives her a prescription, she has it filled without finding out what it is or how it will benefit her. Such people are saying, "I am not worth much."

How do you communicate to a patient that she is worthwhile? Very gently, you help her become aware of what she is doing to herself, because she isn't aware of this. In the past, I made the mistake of saying, "You act as if you aren't worth much," and then the patient became even more ashamed. We need to help her become aware without embarrassing her. We show our patients that they are worthwhile by appreciating and telling them their good qualities.

I want my patients to decide, "I am taking charge," "I'm going to do something about this lupus," "I'm not going to suffer needlessly or feel fated or selected for suffering or victimization."

The greatest tool a healer has is the ability to listen attentively and compassionately to the patient's story. Care-givers who support people's own efforts, who are present with them, give them courage. Physicians should encourage patients to look for what is helpful for them, and encourage them to ask questions and seek answers. Progress is realized little by little, a step at a time. Caretakers and patients work together, using every tool we have.

Dr. Press is an internist in private practice in Monterey, California.

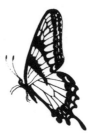

22

Research On Lupus
Interview: David Wofsy, M.D.

Although I am a cautious person, I can't overstate my scientific excitement about what is now being discovered in research on lupus and other immunological diseases.

In the past fifteen years, there have been striking advances in understanding the immune system. We know how it works and what the cells are doing when they make a normal immune response to protect against infection. We also know what is going on when the cells make an abnormal response that contributes to diseases such as lupus. We have learned much more about the molecules that contribute to immune function than was known when the current therapies for autoimmune diseases were being developed.

The current therapies, such as Prednisone and Cytoxan, were based on the fact that, until recently, it was necessary to poison the immune system in order to suppress autoimmune responses. Now our understanding of the immune system is sufficiently sophisticated that we can identify the unique quality of cells, and selectively affect their functions without destroying the entire immune system.

In the laboratory we use a special breed of mice that develop systemic lupus similar to human lupus. It is more common and more severe in female mice, begins in early adulthood, is characterized by the same array of antibodies, and if left untreated is ultimately fatal because of kidney disease.

We are manipulating these strains of mice to learn which cells are important in the development of lupus. Ten years ago we began selectively eliminating various types of cells from the immune system. That is how we discovered that the helper

T cell was playing an important role in the disease. If we eliminated it, mice didn't get lupus. If we eliminated it after they already had lupus, they became less sick. That seemed very promising, but we found that the helper T cells were also needed to assure normal immune function. Therefore, eliminating helper T cells makes the immune system less able to fight off infections. This is similar to the effect of immunosuppressive drugs such as Prednisone. However, unlike Prednisone, eliminating helper T cells did not increase the risks of developing cataracts, diabetes, high blood pressure, osteoporosis, etc., that we can expect from long-term steroid use.

Since our original studies of helper T cells, we have learned to manipulate the immune system in a much more delicate way, based on our understanding of the molecules on the cells. We can get the same level of benefit by blocking the function of molecules rather than eliminating cells. When you stop the therapy, the cells are all there, and the immune system functions normally. It looks promising. So far, this strategy has only been tried on patients with rheumatoid arthritis, but I suspect that these studies will lay the groundwork for treating other illnesses, like lupus.

There are other approaches being explored for the treatment of lupus. We know that there are receptors on the surface of immune cells that recognize and react to antigens (foreign proteins). They also interact with each other. Certain interactions on the molecular level may permit the immune system to attack its own body. It is now possible in the laboratory to block the pathological signal that causes this attack, without causing cell injury.

We want to be able to intervene at a critical point, during a flare of the disease, to turn off the pathological process and achieve a long-lasting effect, so that attacks against the body do not occur for months or years after treatment.

This approach circumvents our ignorance about why the body is making the wrong response. Instead, it may be sufficient to know how to stop the response by blocking distinct molecular interactions. Clinical trials are already showing positive results against psoriasis, another autoimmune disease. With psoriasis it is easy to see almost immediately which treatments work or don't work, so it is possible to fine-tune the medicines used.

Now we think we have some reasonable grounds for making a judgement about the right way to give medicines to effect the cellular responses we want, and it is time to try them on lupus patients. Up to now, we at UCSF (the University of California at San Francisco) have been doing laboratory research, but not clinical trials. We are now about to have a new facility and will begin clinical trials with lupus patients, probably in a cooperative research program with Stanford University. We have a lot of exciting things to try out.

Clinical research in lupus is difficult. Among other things, economic and political factors are involved. For example, as a result of political clout, money has been made available for research and development of products for AIDS and breast cancer. Thus far, no such pressure has been mounted for lupus research.

The profit motive also plays a role. Universities do the basic research, but pharmaceutical companies choose which potential products to develop. They want products they can market profitably, and that is more difficult in lupus than in many other illnesses.

Clinical research in lupus is also difficult because manifestations of the disease are so variable. One person has kidney disease, another has effusions in the lungs, etc. With such different symptoms, it is difficult to design specific clinical trials.

Another obstacle to research is finding appropriate candidates for research. Many people with lupus do not have life-threatening organ involvement, but are clearly compromised by their chronic symptoms of pain and fatigue. With such patients, you have to weigh the risks of experimental treatment against any potential benefits.

Earlier, you asked me to guess about what causes lupus. I don't know anyone who professes to know with certainty. There is a lot of loose talk about stress and the immune system, but there is no convincing scientific evidence that stress can injure the immune system and thereby cause lupus. In fact, what I think is striking is the immune system's ability to withstand assaults of all kinds, including stress. I believe that stress may exacerbate lupus symptoms, but I don't know the mechanism.

Patients ask, "What did I do to bring this on myself?" I don't believe in the notion that people bring on their own diseases, or have lupus because of anything they did. For example, if you already have lupus, sun exposure makes it worse, but sun exposure doesn't cause lupus. In order to get lupus, you probably needed a genetic predisposition, which we don't understand yet and, in addition, you had to encounter the wrong thing, and we don't know what that wrong thing is.

I can't tell you how many positive, optimistic, mentally healthy people I have seen in my career in medicine who have died of cancer or have been very ill with lupus. The idea of mind over matter as a means of controlling serious illness is contrary to my experience.

A positive, enthusiastic attitude toward life, even though it doesn't cure cancer or lupus, lets you make the best of your life.

There is so much we don't know about diseases. It is easy for us, looking back at the medical practices of fifty years ago, to accept that people didn't know everything at that time, and yet we act as if we should know everything right now. Fifty or one hundred years from now, people will not be surprised that we didn't know everything. We are somewhere in the middle of the flow of knowledge, not at the end of it.

Dr. Wofsy is a research physician and professor of Medicine and Microbiology/Immunology at the University of California at San Francisco, and Chief of Rheumatology/Immunology at the Veterans' Administration Medical Center.

MORE RESEARCH NEWS

Northwestern Memorial Hospital in Evanston, Illinois, reports a new process for treating extremely ill lupus patients. It takes stem cells that grow into bone marrow cells, a foundation of the immune system, from a patient's blood, and purifies them. Intense chemotherapy destroys the patient's immune system, and then the purified cells are returned to blossom and recreate the immune system.

Many teaching hospitals are collecting data from lupus patients and their families to identify genetic factors, and also are focusing on possible environmental influences. If you live in the vicinity of a teaching hospital, inquire about research. You may be able to participate in a research study. Often they provide free medication.

Reseachers at the Kitasato Institute in Japan are getting good results in their study of licorice root as a partial substitute for steroids.

Research all over the world continues in an effort to find better medical treatment and even cures for lupus.

23

Let Your Imagination Work For You

Imagery is a very useful tool for dealing with pain and illness, and it doesn't cost a cent. You don't need prescriptions or appointments or long car trips to doctors' offices. Imagery isn't a substitute for any of the drugs and treatment you need, but it's a pleasant way to give yourself some moments of mental well-being. In this chapter you'll learn how to improve your skills at imagining, and then, in the following chapters, you will use these skills to ease your pain, take charge of your own thoughts and images, reduce your worries, and entertain yourself. When life is painful or depressing, a good imagination can give you "time outs" that lift your spirits.

Some people are visually oriented and have no trouble creating internal motion pictures. They see scenes in wonderful technicolor, and envision friends from the past and places they have been, as clearly as if they were there now. Other people can do this only occasionally. They may have trouble seeing old scenes but can invent objects or moving colors when they shut their eyes. Some people visualize only in black and white. Some never see anything that isn't actually there; their "mind's eye" deals in words and thoughts rather than images.

Some people imagine sounds more easily than sights. Beethoven, even when deaf, could hear whole symphonies, whereas many people cannot imagine sound at all. If you are very lucky, you can see in your imagination Beethoven or the Beatles, and at the same time hear their music. You can hear a waltz and imagine a fantastic ballroom filled with costumed dancers, bending and gliding to the music. You can enjoy hearing and seeing samba dancers or imagining picnickers at a cherry blossom festival in Japan.

Some people can smell frying chicken or tacos any time they choose, and others don't imagine smells. Can you remember and recreate in your senses the fragrance of a pine forest or new-cut grass?

Can you recreate in your imagination the taste of chocolate or perhaps a mint julep?

Some people imagine the touch of a caressing hand or a warm summer wind on their skin. They can actually cause temperature changes in their hands or feet by imagining that their hands or feet are in pans of hot water or are wrapped in hot towels. They can cool themselves by imaging ice packs on their foreheads or snow falling softly around them.

Now it is time to play with fantasies. Here are some exercises to sharpen your skill at creating imaginary sights, sounds, smells, tastes, and touch. The exercises are for fun, and to help you expand your powers of imagination.

First, put yourself in a comfortable position. You might sit in your favorite chair or lie in bed with pillows supporting your knees and arms. You might want to place this book on a pillow, so that its weight won't bother you. Begin by letting go any thoughts of the past or future, and be in the present.

Become aware of your breathing. Feel the slight movement of your chest and abdomen as you breathe in and out slowly. Breathe in, hold the air in your lungs for a moment or two, and then purse your lips and make a shhh sound as the air leaves your body. As you breathe out, let your body relax.

We will start with a pear and a plate. To do all of these exercises, you'll need to read a few sentences of explanation, and then close your eyes to do what is suggested. Afterwards, open your eyes again to read further.

Now close your eyes and imagine a bright yellow pear on a bright blue plate. As with all the exercises, open your eyes whenever you choose. Did you imagine that pear and that plate? If not, let yourself experiment. See the color yellow in any way that is possible for you. Then see blue and yellow. Get them arranged into pear and plate. If you cannot see the pear and the plate, think them. That is perfectly all right.

Sometimes an exercise will be easy for you and sometimes you may not be able to do it all. Always, if you can't do it, think it. Everyone can think of the shape of a pear and the shape of a plate, and can think of the colors, even without actually seeing them.

When you are done imagining a yellow pear on a blue plate, let the plate disappear as you imagine that you are holding the pear in one of your hands. Hold the pear in front of you as you imagine its weight and smooth coolness. See its yellowness.

Lift the pear to your nose and sniff the pear fragrance. Feel your mouth grow moist even before your pear touches your lips. Even before you bite into your pear, your mouth is ready. Feel how moist and ready your mouth becomes. Experience your lips against the cool pear. Bite the pear and feel your teeth against the cool pear, and feel the cool softness of the pear in your mouth. Taste the sweet soft pear-taste in your mouth. Be aware of this delicate taste as you chew and then swallow. Look at the pear again and see the moist whiteness where you took a bite. Take another bite if you like, chew, swallow, and when you are ready, stop imagining a pear. Let it disappear from your hand.

Another exercise. In reality, you can no longer sit in the sun on a beach, because sun is dangerous for anyone with lupus, but you can pretend to be there. Imagine that you are lying on a hammock between two palm trees on a white sand beach. The hammock is red. The tops of the palm trees are green. In front of you, you see the bright blue ocean and the foamy, white crests of the waves breaking against the white sand. The sky is blue. If you like, you can imagine people walking by. Perhaps it is a Mexican beach, with Mexican venders holding bouquets of huge, bright paper flowers or many-colored serapes. It can be any beach you choose. Stay in the hammock as long as you like.

When you are finished imagining your beach, get ready for some silliness. Stay on the bright red hammock, and this time imagine a chocolate beach. See the brown color and smell the chocolate. Rolling in toward you are vanilla waves on a strawberry sea. What color is your sky? Candy-striped? Mint green?

Imagine a funky plaid beach with matching hammock, lavender water and green sky. Imagine orange sand and a deep purple sea and a polka-dot sky. What wonders you can make inside your head!

Occasionally, someone finds that her fantasy becomes unpleasant. You might be enjoying the orange sand and purple see, when suddenly you give yourself the image of a monster or a hurricane in the distance. If you have that type of rebellious imagination, move outside of your fantasy and become an observer, who watches the person in the hammock and the monster or hurricane. As observer, you'll learn that you can allow yourself fantasy nightmares without feeling frightened or hurt. If you follow the fantasy to its conclusion, you learn some useful information about yourself.

When you are ready, imagine that Aladdin's genie approaches your hammock, sprinkles it with diamond-colored sand, and turns it into a flying carpet that you control. Feel the hammock slowly untie itself from the palm trees and rise in the air. If you like such a trip, you and your hammock can soar high over the palms. You can fly all over the world on your hammock. If you prefer a more conservative ride, imagine that you are floating slowly, two feet above the sand. Put a peephole in your hammock and see brightly-colored fish in the water.

And now it is time to hear music. If you have difficulty hearing music that is not there, start with the simple song that you knew when you were a child, "Twinkle, twinkle little star."

To get started, hum it to yourself, then stop humming and imagine a little child singing it to you. Now hear a deep, alto voice singing the song. Add cellos or bagpipes or trumpets or flutes, whatever you prefer. Make the sounds silly or sweet. A huge orchestra may be playing the song.

Imagine yourself a little child singing to the tune of "Twinkle, twinkle":

"Guess what, guess what I can do.

I hear music, you can too."

If you don't quite hear it, think the words.

Would you like to listen to the sound of leaves rustling in the wind, or water flowing in a creek? Imagine your special hammock between two pine trees, deep in a lovely wooded forest. On the ground are violets, little irises, bright green grass, and perhaps a bed of four-leaf clovers. A breeze blows softly against your face, and last year's leaves make a dry, crinkling sound.

Now imagine a stream flowing beside your hammock. You can hear its music as it tumbles between small rocks. Do you hear the birds in the trees? Stay in this scene as long as you please, and then come back.

When you are back in your room, let yourself notice your real surroundings. Pretend that you are in your room for the first time, and examine it with excitement. Do you have attractive wallpaper in your room, a glass vase that reflects light, a family photo you especially like, or a painting? Find objects to notice, just as if the room were new to you. Perhaps you can see a tree outside your window. Look at it carefully and enjoy its color, shape, size, and texture.

Next, notice what you can hear. Perhaps it is raining, and you hear the ping of the raindrops against your window. Do you hear your refrigerator humming, or cars honking? What else do you hear?

Are you aware of fragrances? Can you smell flowers or cooking odors or the pungent smell of dirt after rain?

Now feel the softness of the pillow that cradles your head, the texture of the chair or bedding against your arms and buttocks. Even if your hands are hurting, let them touch each other very softly, and experience the feeling of two hands caring for each other.

Perhaps it is time to have a real cup of herb tea or a piece of fruit. Enjoy. Remember that you can always look for pleasure where you are, or you can use your imagination to go to other times and other places.

In the next chapter you will learn how to combine your imagination and your awareness of your breathing to ease your aches and bring you serenity. After that, you'll use your power of positive imagination to claim your autonomy and reduce your worries.

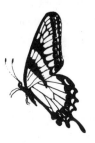

24

Breathe Your Way to Serenity

Even when life is difficult and pain is sharp, you can still breathe tenderly into your body. You can breathe in loving air and imagine it caressing the places that ache.

First, get comfortable. If you haven't already learned the importance of soft pillows, beg, borrow or buy lots of them and place them in different positions until you have found a way to rest your body luxuriously.

When you are as comfortable as possible, put your hands on your abdomen just below your belly button, so that you can feel your abdomen rise and fill as you breathe in. Let the air remain a moment or two in your lungs, and then feel your abdomen sink as you expel the air from your lungs. Breathe deeply, slowly, and naturally.

With each breath relax one part of your body: feet, ankles, knees, thighs, hips, abdomen, stomach, chest, shoulders, arms, hands, throat, neck, head, face, jaw. The way to do this is simple. Breathe in naturally, and as you breathe out relax one part of your body. Start with your feet. After they are relaxed, breathe again, then exhale and relax your ankles. Keep breathing slowly and evenly as you relax each part of your body in turn.

When your body is relaxed, you can tackle the spots that give you special trouble. These are the places that ache, sting, or simply stay tight. For these spots, you will change your concentration slightly. Instead of relaxing your body as you exhale, this time you'll pay attention to what you do before you exhale.

As you breathe in slowly and deeply, imagine that a healing air is flowing through your nose to your lungs and on to a part of your body that is hurting you. Imagine that this air cleanses and begins to heal that hurting spot. When you breathe out slowly, the air leaves your body through your mouth, taking hurts and impurities with it. Inhale the healing air through your nose, and exhale the impurities through your mouth.

Imagine that you are sending this healing air to your internal organs, your liver, heart, brain, as well as any other part of you that might need healing. Breathe in slowly and deeply, and let yourself relax.

That is as much concentration on breathing as you are likely to want to do in one session. You can return to this exercise whenever you like. Remember always to let yourself breathe in a slow, natural, relaxed way.

Now you will begin to combine breathing awareness with imaginary adventures. As you lie on your pillows or sit comfortably in your chair, imagine that you are walking along a stone path. On either side are dozens of beautiful bushes, with exotic, many colored flowers. Ahead of you is a magic castle, with a large, carved stone door. As you approach, the door opens slowly. Go inside.

The first thing you see inside the castle is a huge room with a long table filled with rows of fancy bottles. In these bottles are unending supplies of magical, colored air for you to breathe. There are cut-glass bottles with pink air, and tiny bottles with etchings of flowers that contain a soft blue air. Every imaginable bottle is there in front of you on the long table.

Pick one up, and notice that it uncaps itself. The colored air rises from the bottle and moves gently toward your face. You face feels soft, because it is being bathed in this lovely air. As you breathe it in, this magic air goes to your sore joints, or wherever you choose.

Because the number of bottles is unending and each bottle re-fills itself even before it is emptied, you can keep breathing the essences of the magic air for as long as you like. Perhaps you will fall asleep surrounded by beautiful colored air.

On another trip into the castle, go past the table with bottles into another room. Here you will find a very special, magic lamp, hanging from a peg in the stone wall. Take the lamp off the peg, and shine it toward any part of your body that needs magic relief. Its soft pink light will focus on the places that hurt.

In another room you may discover an air throne, made of millions of colored air bubbles that hold you tenderly, as it relaxes you and relieves your pain.

Perhaps deep in the castle in an almost hidden corner, you discover a little shop with a sign "Magic For Sale" in the window. Inside is a proprietor, a sorcerer with brown or black or white skin, and happy robes of brilliant colors. You tell the proprietor what is hurting you today, and the proprietor mixes a special salve and offers it to you in a tiny gold box. Dip one finger in the salve and touch your finger to any part of your body that is giving you discomfort. As you breathe in and out, slowly and deeply, the salve seems to light up your skin and comforts your aches.

You may imagine that you discover a pool deep inside the castle. You decide to undress and enter the warm water, and as you float, music plays and healing perfume fills the air.

These are a few samples of the ways in which you can combine breathing and imagining. If you have young children or grandchildren, you can tell them stories about visiting such happy places as magic castles with bottles of colored air, hidden pools, and wise people who will answer their questions or give them salves. Whenever you like, you can invent new stories for yourself.

Occasionally some people feel as if they can't control their fantasies. Instead of health-giving, beautiful scenes, something goes wrong. The magic castle is ugly or the wise person is foolish. If this happens to you, don't fight against yourself. Instead, be the observer who watches you within your fantasy.

See what you can learn from any unhappy shift in the fantasy. Often, there is an important reason you are not letting yourself be comforted, and that reason may have real significance for you. When you are ready, either go back to a happy fantasy or do something else that would be pleasant for you.

Now that you have learned to concentrate on slow, deep breathing while using your powers to imagine, you will discover that you don't have to lie down to visit your own magic castle or breathe in healing air. As you drive, you can pretend you are on the air-throne or in a pool. You can imagine inhaling mellow, healing air, no matter where you are or what you are doing.

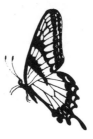

25

Choose Who May Live In Your Head

Lupus is a disease that can be devastating to you. It may force you to quit work. It may drive away friends and lovers who run from the reality of your illness. Your children may have to live elsewhere temporarily, because you are too ill to care for them. The medicines you need to combat lupus may have bad side effects, or even cause other illnesses. Feelings of depression and despair may be a natural reaction to your setbacks and losses or may be caused by the disease itself or the medicines you have to take. So these truths could seem like a bad joke:

You are in charge of your behavior.

You are in charge of your feelings.

You are in charge of your beliefs and thoughts.

They make more sense when you add: Although you are not able to be in charge of your lupus, you are in charge of your behavior, thoughts, and feelings about it.

Expanding your sense of autonomy will help you become less victimized by your illness and therefore happier about yourself. This chapter will show you ways in which you can recognize and develop your sense of personal autonomy.

You are in charge of your behavior. A persuasive salesperson may try to make you buy a new car, but you still decide to buy or not to buy. When you clean your house, whether in response to your belief that you must do it or in response to your partner's belief that it's your job, you are the one who is responsible for your actions. No one makes you clean the house. If you decide, "I am too tired to clean the house so I will rest today," you are responsible for that behavior, too. There are many behavioral choices you make every day, and most of them are neither right nor wrong. They are merely the behaviors you choose. In the long run, you will be much happier when you recognize that. It doesn't work well for people to believe that fate or other people make them do the things you do.

Practice autonomous behavior by answering, "What is my reason for choosing to do what I am about to do?" For example, "I am choosing to go to work today, even though I am sick." Remind yourself, "I don't have to go to work, even if I will suffer financially by staying home. I can make arrangements to stay home when I am sick, I can quit work, I can ask for part-time work. At this point in my life, I am choosing to go to work."

At your mother's home, you are offered a piece of pie. Remind yourself, "I don't have to eat it just because she baked it. I am choosing to eat a piece of pie. I also choose whether to enjoy it or feel guilty about the calories in the pie."

You are in charge of your emotions. No one can make you feel. If a tiger walked through the front door into your living room this minute, you would be terrified because you know that tigers are dangerous. You are the one who knows that, not the tiger. You, not the tiger, are the one who gives you the message to be afraid. A very small child might say "Big Kitty" and run happily to the tiger. You are in charge of your feelings, and your feelings depend on your own way of labeling people, places, and events. You choose your feelings about your lupus, as well as your feelings about everything else.

The only thing in life that you can really control is your attitude.

For instance, if you tell yourself that life with lupus is not worth living, you may make yourself depressed and even suicidal. If you remind yourself of some pleasures you experienced yesterday or today, you make yourself less depressed.

Sometimes you'll choose to remember pleasures and sometimes you'll want to let yourself feel your sorrows and pain.

The fact that you are in charge of your feelings, doesn't mean that you must paste a phoney smile on your face. You may choose to storm, sob, sulk, or shiver. Sometimes you choose to smile even though you know your honest response would be to groan. Other times you choose to groan. The next chapter deals more thoroughly with emotions and what to do about them.

You are in charge of your beliefs and thoughts. No one but you can create your thoughts. When you choose to clean your house "because company is coming," you are the one who thinks up that reason, even if you heard this command first from your mother or grandmother. You and only you are responsible for maintaining the belief that you must clean for company, instead of listening to your body, when it says, "Not today, because today I am exhausted!"

When you wake up in the morning, remembering an idea that seemed to come in your sleep, it is you who thought up the idea and then remembered it. The idea wasn't zapped into your brain. When you decide to believe something that one of the women in your lupus support group tells you, you are the one who does the believing. She can't "make you believe."

As you read the section of this book, "lupus club members tell their stories," you noticed how very differently each person thought about events in her life. You probably argued in your head with some of the thoughts and beliefs, and agreed with others. That is always your choice.

Sometimes your mind clouds or gets off track, from medication or the disease itself. It's hard to straighten out drug-induced or disease-induced thoughts. Still, even your crazy thoughts are your own. They may be the only thoughts you are able to think at that moment.

There are also irrational thoughts that do not come from drugs or illness. They come from what we learn and mis-learn while growing up. Too often, these thoughts are self-critical and hurtful. We give them to ourselves when we think we've done something wrong or stupid or even slightly less than perfect. Sometimes it may feel as if there is a war going on inside your brain between your healthy sense of yourself and your self-criticism. If you listen carefully to yourself, you even wonder:

WHO IS LIVING IN MY HEAD?

The answer: You, like everyone else, have a whole cast of characters up there in the gray matter, heroes and cowards, thinkers and dopes, helpers and villains, friends and enemies. You collected yours in childhood and have been adding to the list ever since. These voices may clutter up your mind and leave you unhappy. You may have become so accustomed to your villains that you scarcely notice how they damage your self-esteem.

Once you get to know your own cast of characters, you can sort them out, in order to enjoy your heroes and stop listening to your villains. Getting to know these characters is interesting and fun.

One way to know the villains in your own head is to recreate a scene in which they are most likely to pop out. For example, when was the last time you mislaid something, an important letter or your car keys or your purse? Remember the scene and put yourself back into it. Listen to what you are saying to yourself.

"You stupid klutz! You lose everything!"

"You must be going crazy, forgetting things the way you do!"

"You never put things were they belong!"

"You never do anything right!"

"This is a disaster! Probably someone has already found your purse, read your address inside it, and right this minute is ransacking your home."

"It's the kids' fault. If they hadn't gotten you so riled up, you'd know where you put the keys."

"Is lupus making you loose your mind!"

Are any of these villains among your cast of characters? If so, notice that they are worse than worthless. These internal enemies distract you from your search for whatever you mislaid, while causing you tension and misery. They inhibit your ability to think. They keep you chronically sad, angry, frightened, or ashamed. You don't deserve such villains messing about inside your head. They have probably been there for so many years that you have grown accustomed to them, and never even considered that you can live without them.

You can't control what other people in your life say to you, but you can control what you say to yourself. That is what autonomy is all about.

Test out one more scene. You are at your doctor's office. It took some effort to get there, and now, unfortunately, you discover that your scheduled appointment was for yesterday, not today. You made a mistake, and today your doctor is not in the office. You are disappointed, but you make another appointment with the receptionist, apologize, and leave.

Which of your villains gets on your case? Imagine the scene, and listen carefully to what goes on in your head. Perhaps you bully yourself, telling yourself you are stupid or worthless. Or do you hear a "Nervous Nellie," worrying you about what the doctor will think of you because you forgot the appointment? Perhaps you have in your head a Pseudo-Comforter, who tells you, "Never mind, nobody with lupus can be expected to remember dates." That one doesn't help, either.

Would you like to get rid of your villains? It's easy to do.

Go back to a scene such as the one in the doctor's office, or use a scene in which you are searching for something you mislaid. Hear the words your villain uses against you.

In the past, you may have tried to argue with these voices. Never do that. It doesn't work. Instead, bring silliness and humor to the task of villain-zapping. First, listen again to the words your villain uses, and then pretend an actor in a TV drama is speaking those lines. How might such a villain look? Dress your villain as ridiculously as you like, and give him or her a name.

For example, you may name your villain, Barney the Blamer. He may have a tiny, round face, wear an orange and purple pin-striped, three-piece suit, and waggle his finger at you as he scolds, "Why can't you ever keep track of anything? You are always losing things!" Those words, "why can't you ever" and "you are always" are stupid exaggerations, so you dressed him to fit his exaggerated stupidity.

You may name your villain Wilma the Witch, and dress her in a black robe and pointed hat. Give her a long nose and put a purple wart on the end of it. Her witchy comments were, "You'll never find the keys, because you never find anything!" That is a ridiculous curse, isn't it?

Have fun naming and dressing your villain.

Imagine your villain on your TV screen. Your villain is shuffling or leaping about, gesturing and yelling. As you watch and listen, notice how boring the words are. Increase the speed, so that the villain is speaking faster and faster until all the words run together into one thin squeak. Slow the speed, and listen as the words go from squeak to grunt. As you change the speed, you'll notice that your villain's gestures and facial expressions whirl and then slow into sodden absurdity.

Watch your villain drool or get red-faced or fall on its face. When you are tired of listening to the villain, press Mute. You can watch your villain, mouth open, screeching silently. Don't hurry through this fantasy. Relax and enjoy it. After all, you've suffered for years from listening to your own self-scolding. Now is the time to make the scolding comic.

Turn off the TV, if you like, and pretend you are the villain. Speak the words, but put the emPHAsis on the wrong syLLABLEs. Make up a silly accent. Or say the words without moving your tongue.

Put your villain back on TV, and practice making the villain disappear and appear again with an imaginary click of the power button. Whenever you hear yourself scolding you, put the scolding part of yourself on TV, listen awhile, play with the images and sounds, and then practice turning the power on and off. You are in charge!

People sometimes forget that their fantastic brains are, like TV sets, equipped not only with an off/on switch but also a channel selector. List a few alternate channels: "My Vacations," "Happy Memories," "Home Comedies," as well as your own private X-rated film, "Love With My Sweetheart." You have hundreds of channels in your brain. Turn on your imaginary TV and practice changing channels.

You are proving to yourself that you are in charge of your own brain. Many people, including famous psychotherapists, do not know that people control their own minds. They say, "A thought came to me." (From outer space?) Or they say, "I can't help thinking about ...." They offer fraudulent experiments, such as, "Try not to think of a pink elephant," and then nod wisely when you agree that you are thinking of the elephant.

Pretend you are in a swing, and you are just old enough to have learned to pump the swing by yourself. Stretch out your legs and pull back on the ropes, and up you go! Pull back again and stretch your legs and swing higher. And down and then up, and down and up again. The breeze blows your hair, your stomach tingles, and you laugh as you swing so high and free.

Are you still with the psychotherapist's elephant? Of course not. You stopped trying NOT to think, and, instead, simply changed channels. So easy!

However, because your villains have been part of your life for years, you may find them back in your head from time to time. You can use lots of fun tricks to defeat the villains in your brain.

Use a sparkling, diamond-studded, anti-villain wand that is hanging invisibly on the kitchen wall. Any time you begin to scold yourself, wave your magic wand and, poof, the villain disappears.

Perhaps you prefer an anti-villain spray can filled with villain-repellant.

Send your villain on a one-way trip to Mars.

Have you got the idea? If so, you now are ready to demolish your worst internal villains, the enemies who attack you in the most vulnerable parts of your being.

About your lupus rash: "You are so ugly that no one will ever love you," or "The way you look, who would want to marry you?"

About your pain and exhaustion: "Maybe the doctors are right that you are a hypochondriac," or "If you weren't such a weakling, you wouldn't let lupus get you down."

About your kidneys: "If you had taken better care of yourself, this wouldn't be happening to you," or "You're going to lose your kidneys and it's your own fault."

About your depression: "Just snap out of it and stop being a baby."

If you try to out-argue these hurtful voices, you won't win. Arguing against self-destructive thoughts is in itself stressful. The easiest way to rid yourself of these self-inflicted hurts is to make fun of them.

The voice says, "You are too ugly for anyone to love." It's a crazy message, but arguing internally about it will not help much. Instead, imagine a super-ugly witch, warts everywhere, jealously telling you that. Then let the voice whine, squeak, become unintelligible. Throw water on the hag, and watch her melt to nothing, as Dorothy did in the Oz story. Switch channels. Perhaps right now a religious channel would be comforting for you. Or switch off the internal TV and call a friend. Or plan where to go to meet new friends.

Of course it's not your fault that your lupus has invaded your kidneys. If there is something you can do that will help your kidneys, you'll do it. Torturing yourself with words is never helpful. So put the voice on TV and then press mute. Better yet, pretend the voice is coming from a nasty little bug. Step on it, squashing it into the carpet.

About your pain and exhaustion - - listening to criticism is also exhausting, and depressing. Why in the world would you keep someone like that inside your head? Put your internal enemy on a special rocket jet, light a magic fuse, and watch as the jet, with the enemy inside, goes whizzing out your window toward Mars.

Practice any crazy way at all of getting rid of the enemies in your own head.

In place of villains, you need admirers and friends, internal voices that cherish you. First, find an admirer, someone who is proud of you. For example, a boy named Brian got a very special report card in the third grade: "Brian consistently works with great effort and performs with excellence. He is a fine citizen and a very special part of our class." That teacher knew the importance of praise!

You need such people in your head. Their voices can help you feel proud of the way you are coping with a terrible disease. Remember someone from your childhood who admired you. If you don't think of anyone, invent an admirer. Write a note to yourself, like the note Brian received.

In addition to admirers, you need internal friends. A friend likes you just the way you are, listens to you, and enjoys you. Friends are pals who let you know that you are an interesting, likeable human being. A friend doesn't try to change you. Make a list of past and present pals in your life. Take in any happy, friendly words they have said to you, and keep those words in your memory. If you don't have enough pals in your present life, join a lupus support group. You'll find them there.

Your pets are pals, who love you just the way you are. When you find yourself listening to unhappy messages, one good piece of advice is to hug your pet.

Besides friends and admirers, you need voices in your head that are wise, nurturing, and caring. You might start by inventing your own personal fairy godmother. Don't use Cinderella's. That old lady made a carriage and a pretty dress for Cinderella, but did she really help Cinderella feel OK about herself without all the finery? Did she let Cinderella know that she could tell people firmly, "I am not cleaning the hearth today," and still be a worthwhile human being? Unfortunately, unless Cinderella found herself a better fairy godmother or parent to put in her head, she probably ended up sad and overworked, cleaning the prince's hearths almost as soon as the honeymoon was over!

Imagine for yourself a wise Fairy Godmother whose loving will be right for you. Hear her say, "I love you." "You are valuable." "You are lovable." "You are good." "You are important." "I want you to take good care of yourself." You can teach your personal fairy godmother to whisper these magic words to you whenever you wish.

Find your own memories from your childhood. If you were lucky, you remember lots of scenes of being held, kissed, and spoken to with love by parents and relatives. Grab every loving person and loving scene you can remember, and keep them in your head. They are wonderful substitutes for the villains you are tossing out. If you don't remember loving people in your childhood, invent them. For models you can use loving people from books, movies, or real life. Practice parenting yourself lovingly whenever you are tired or hurting, as well as when you feel well and are happy. A loving parent in your head is beautiful medicine.

Every loving image you keep in your head becomes a part of you. Practice loving yourself.

Getting rid of your villains and substituting self-approval, self-caring, and self-love can be done alone or in groups. In lupus groups, members laugh and support each other, as villains are zapped. Supporting others and being supported, while learning to love oneself, is a beautiful and powerful group experience.

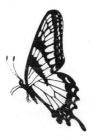

26

Accept Your Feelings

When members of a local lupus support group decided to start a writing group, this is what Rialta (chapter 4) wrote:

"This morning a soft, lovely fog envelops the world outside my window. Even my trees have vanished. There are no street sounds, just white mist, silence, and peacefulness. I lie on my couch, talking into a recording machine. My hands hurt too much to use them for typing today, but I will type this later.

"I am remembering what I used to do ... run up and down the hills in fog and sun, happy as a puppy, type easily, aspire to an advanced degree and a fascinating job.

"This quiet morning I do not want to struggle into happiness. I want to lie right here, and mourn the health I no longer have. I want to mourn the babies I will never have. I want to rage against tiredness and pain."

Emotional health doesn't mean perpetual happiness. It means the ability to experience and accept a full range of feelings, without being trapped by any one feeling. In our society, there are lots of crazy beliefs that prevent easy access to our feelings. Here are a few of them: Don't be too happy, or something bad will happen. A few tears may be acceptable, but too many tears are shameful. Sighs are acceptable, but anger is not lady-like. Fear is childish, and should be hidden. "Smile and the world smiles with you. Weep and you weep alone."

Some people, who learned in childhood that their feelings were intolerable to their parents, spend a lifetime attempting to mute or discount their feelings.

All of us look at the world through the lenses of early childhood experiences. We react as we were taught to react when we were young. Want to check this out? Here is an exercise to help you remember what you learned about feelings when you were a child. Test out each emotion separately:

Imagine that you are five years old. You are about to run inside the house or apartment where you live. The rest of your family is inside.

You've fallen and scraped your knee. It is bleeding and it hurts. Run inside, crying, and show everyone your knee and tell them it hurts. What are their responses?

Run into the house, sad and crying, because you lost your pet turtle, or your best friend is moving away.

Run in angrily, shouting that a big kid stole your cookie from your lunch box.

Again, run in angrily. Tell your mother that she made you the kind of sandwich you hate, and she forgot to put a cookie in your lunch box.

Run in scared. You thought you saw something big and awful behind the house.

Walk in slowly, with your lower lip pouting. You are jealous, because your best friend got something you wish you had, like a better grade or an invitation to a birthday party.

You are ashamed. While you were running home, you wet your pants.

Run in laughing and happy. You got the A or the invitation to a party.

Run in laughing and happy for no reason at all. You feel good all over.

As you imagine the facial expressions and the responses from the various people in your family, you'll know which emotions are accepted and which are rejected or ignored in your house.

In therapy you might explore these scenes, as you relate them to your current experiences with showing feeling. You can also explore them by yourself in order to get to know yourself better. Whether or not you explore these scenes more thoroughly, it is important to give yourself permission to know your emotions and to share them with others.

Go back into the imaginary scenes, when you are five years old and about to run inside the house or apartment where you live. The rest of your family is no longer there. Instead, you, an adult, are in their place. You will offer the five-year-old the love and acceptance she needed back then. Alternate being the child and being yourself, the adult, and experience the satisfaction of comforting and being comforted.

The child runs in, crying about her hurt knee. You comfort her. Don't rush her through her tears or try to distract her. She has a right to respond to her own hurts in her own way, without anyone else defining them for her. Accept and honor her ability to express her feelings, and give her a band-aid to put on her knee. When she is ready, she'll be happy again. Savor your adult role. This is a way you can treat yourself today, whenever you are hurting. Be the child and take into yourself the love you received.

Let the sad child tell you what was special about her turtle. After her sadness has been heard and accepted, she will decide when to stop being sad. A wise parent listens instead of rushing in to "make everything all right." The next day or the next week, the child may again remember her turtle sadly, and that also is healthy. There is not a mandatory time limit for any grief.

Perhaps in your childhood you were lucky enough to have experienced nothing more traumatic than a lost or dead turtle. However, if there was real tragedy in your childhood, you might want to go back to those scenes to help yourself, as adult and child, express your grief and deal with your tragedy.

Understand the child's fury at the kid who stole the cookie. She has a right to her own anger. Later, the two of you may want to talk about how she can seek protection from the big kids, but right now you are giving her permission to experience her own rage, tell it in her own way, and know that she is being heard.

It is hard to accept a child's anger when you are the target. Be a spectacularly good mother to this youngster, by letting her know that you accept her fury at you for your poor choice of sandwich material and your forgetfulness about cookies, and tell her you're sorry. Remind yourself that in the future you will pay attention to this child's anger, and take better care of her.

Listen to the child's fear of something big and awful. Let her know that fear is a natural response to a perception of danger. Later, you and she can take a flashlight outside to see what is out there.

Lots of children have been taught that it is not "nice" to be jealous, so they try to hide their jealousy. Tell your five-year-old that you understand that she is jealous, and encourage her to say more about it. Don't try to argue her out of any feeling that is hers.

Shame is so difficult an emotion that it requires very special understanding. "It is awful to be ashamed, isn't it?" You'll want to hug her and let her know that she is a wonderful person and, naturally, she feels ashamed about wet pants. Everyone does feel ashamed of this, even though almost everyone in the whole world wets her pants from time to time.

When she races in happy, for whatever reason, the two of you laugh and cheer together.

How will you use these same techniques, empathy and love, toward yourself today? As Rialta wrote, "This quiet morning I do not want to struggle into happiness." Instead, she accepts her sadness, and also her anger at her tiredness and pain. Will you do the same for yourself?

Let yourself know your current sadness and emotional hurt. When you fight your feelings, you attack yourself. Listen to the difference between, "I'm sad right now," and the self-critical, "Oh, damn, here I go again!" or "I've got to stop feeling sorry for myself!" Your sadness is valid simply because it is what you feel. When you've accepted your sadness, choose a compassionate friend and share your feelings with that friend.

If you are chronically sad, you may be stuck in mourning for what you have lost. Lupus patients may have lost homes, income, jobs, health, physical attributes and abilities, goals and objectives, and people who were close to them. Some of your losses may seem insignificant and others may seem almost insurmountable. Each person reacts in her own fashion to her losses.

Give yourself permission to mourn your losses for as long as you choose. When you are ready, you can say good-bye to the past, and to the plans and dreams for a future that cannot come true for you. By letting go of mourning about the past and the future, you can live more fully in the present.

Take your good-byes one at a time, starting with those that are easiest for you. Get comfortable, breathe slowly and deeply, relax your body, and let yourself travel through your memory to a specific scene in which you'll be saying good-bye to some past aspect of your life.

One woman said good-bye to her ability to play competitive tennis. She remembered the time she won an important local tournament, and re-played it in her fantasy. She experienced the thrill of her body's skill and endurance, and was aware of people cheering for her. Then, as the woman she is today, she joined the scene and congratulated herself, the winner. "You were good. And you were me. You are me in the past. And now I am saying good-bye to my ability to play tennis."

Another woman mourned the loss of her tan. To say good-bye, she imagined sitting beside the tanned woman she was. "Your skin is brown and beautiful, and I envy you." She began to laugh, as she remembered how her grandmother had prized her own very white skin. She said aloud, "Well, Grannie, now my skin is like yours. And now I know that skin color is unimportant. I wish the whole world knew this." Then she said good-bye to the tanned girl she once had been.

Many people grieve over lost jobs. To say good-bye to your past employment, create a scene in which you are doing the work you loved. Bring your co-workers into this imaginary scene and talk to them about what you liked and disliked about this job. Take as long as you want, and then imagine that you are saying good-bye to the place and the people. Finish by saying, "Good-bye, job."

Tamara (chapter 13) said about her lover, "We ended our seven- year relationship, which had begun with so much joy and hopefulness. I was sad about that, because a dream had ended." She imagined Patrick and herself together in their home, told him her resentments and appreciations, said good-bye, and imagined him walking away, out of the house and her life. Some months later, she began dating a man who understands her physical problems and is good to her.

After good-byes, memories do remain. Instead of being saddened by them, you can choose to be grateful that once upon a time you could dance until dawn, run easily, type without pain, hold a job you loved. The ability to remember is one of the joys of being human. You stored lovely memories of yourself to cherish whenever you choose.

Good-byes also need to be said for dreams and hopes that never will come true. Some people put in years of study in order to have a profession that their physical damage from lupus has made impossible. Some can never have children. As in other good-byes, pick a hoped-for scene, experience it, know your sorrow that this scene will never come true, and say good-bye to what you can't have. You have a right to mourn your loss for as long as you choose and whenever you choose.

Later, when you are ready, you can think about what you can do to make your present life as fulfilling as possible. Perhaps you don't have the physical stamina for medical school, but you might assist in a medical research laboratory. If you can neither conceive nor care for an infant, perhaps you can find a way to enjoy a pet or someone else's child. Enjoying the present is more worthwhile than mourning an impossible future.

Let yourself be angry. Anger, not expressed, often becomes an unpleasant whining or a hard lump in the stomach. You may need to be truly angry at what has happened to you. Turn up the radio, if you like, so that you won't alarm your neighbors, and yell your fury. That often feels very good. The best things you can do, pounding pillows and kicking them around the house, might cause your joints to ache, so instead, fantasize hitting, scratching, slugging, or stabbing. If you are angry at a person, imagine the most outlandish thing you would like to do. Remember that thoughts and actions are totally different. You can imagine smashing someone's nose with great enjoyment, even though you would never hit anyone.

Jealousy is a natural and universal feeling. Sometimes you may be jealous even of your own children, who are healthy and can go to the beach, while you are stuck indoors. You may be jealous of your pain-free friends and relatives, especially when your body is hurting. If you try to shut away your jealousy, you may find it creeping into all sorts of situations, and turning into crankiness. Better to admit, "I am jealous of every person who can do things I used to enjoy doing!" "I am jealous of everyone who is healthy!" Yell that loudly, if you choose. Then be your own nurturing parent, and give yourself extra kindness and perhaps a small stay-at-home present.

All lupus patients are well-acquainted with fear, as they face difficult medical proceedures, or wonder what tomorrow may bring. You can't force yourself to stop being afraid, nor can you shame your fears away, no matter how hard you try. Trying not to be afraid can even increase your tension, and your pain. You certainly don't need self-scolding or shaming for being afraid. You need to give yourself whatever will help diminish your fear. Whether your fears are real or fantasied, you need some equivalent of a good flashlight!

If you are terrified that your kidneys are beginning to malfunction, get them tested often. If you are afraid that something may be happening to your eyes, have them checked. Insist on having a doctor who understands your fears, and agrees to be truthful at all times about your condition.

Give yourself permission to say, "I'm afraid" to your doctor, nurses, family, and friends, and to ask for the support you need. When you are in the hospital, you'll want someone with you who cares about you, knows your disease, and is capable of explaining to you what is happening. Bring along an "advocate" to speak up for you. No one should have to be alone in the hospital. Members of your lupus support group, who have experienced what you are now facing, can help you with whatever is fearful.

Cheer for yourself whenever you are happy. Little bits of fun will occur even in the worst stages of your illness, and during good cycles you can be happy for days or weeks at a time. Happiness is a welcome gift to yourself. Some women make a list of ways to make themselves happy, and put the list on the bathroom mirror:

Call a cheerful friend

Keep flowers in my house

Ask the librarian for humorous books

Rent a funny video

Buy art supplies and learn to paint

Join a ceramics class, poker club, or bridge group

There are dozens of happy activities. Look for a pleasant, happy, or funny experience each day to store in your memory, but don't berate yourself if on some days nothing is good.

You are not a failure if you act less heroically or less successfully than some lupus patients. Not everyone who is undergoing dialysis has the energy to toss her dialysis bag over the rear-view mirror and drive happily to San Francisco, as Pamela does. Honor your own unique emotional reactions to lupus, without comparing yourself negatively to other lupus sufferers. You'll feel more whole if you permit yourself both joy and tears, without making any emotion a "should."

There may come a time when you are able to say honestly, "I've learned a lot from my experience with lupus, and become a richer person in spite of my illness." You've probably learned patience and self-acceptance, and gained in inner strength. You've experienced bitterness over what you have lost, and guilt when you have to let people down. And you know that neither of these emotions is helpful to you.

You've learned to sort out your feelings, accept them, and let them go. You know how to listen to yourself, befriend yourself, and remind yourself that you are a survivor.

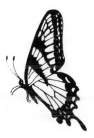

27

Banish Your Worries

Worries are unhappy stories we tell ourselves over and over
again, about a future that may or may not occur. Nothing good comes from worrying. Worry may give us merely a
moment of unease, or it may become an almost constant, self-
inflicted torment. Worry increases our fatigue; as one member
of the lupus support group said, "I am sick and tired of being
sick and tired, and the more I worry the more sick and tired I
become."

Worrying produces feelings of fear, shame, self-doubt, self-
hate, internal tension, and depression. It may activate headaches, insomnia, or asthma attacks, elevate blood pressure to
dangerous levels, and perhaps trigger lupus flares. When tension from worry leads to physical distress, it seems as if worry
causes the very conditions that the individual worries about.

When you have lupus, it is difficult not to worry. Lupus is
a crazy, inconsistent illness, with flares, remissions, and unpredictable symptoms that spring up overnight. Even if you were
not a worrier before you had lupus, when you suffer from lupus
it's easy to become one. There are dozens of lupus-triggered
worries.

"I worry that my lover will become tired of my sickness
and leave me." "I worry that no one will ever ask me for dates,
because of the rash on my face." "I worry that my kidneys will
fail, and I'll need to go on dialysis." "What if I get a bowel
obstruction and end up with a colostomy?" "If I can't go on
working, what will happen to me?" "I worry that my being
sick is affecting my children badly." "I worry that I won't be
able to pay my bills."

Unlike the disease of lupus, the pseudo-disease of worry is curable. Even the most intractable worrier can learn to stop worrying.

There are different types of worries, and each type needs to be dealt with in a different manner. Whenever you begin to worry, ask yourself:

Am I worrying about something trivial?

Trivial worries are those that, even if they do come true, won't matter much in a person's life. Vera's (chapter 9) worry about getting her Christmas cards written on time is a trivial worry.

Is my worry about something that won't happen?

Worries can be classified in terms of their likelihood of coming true. Beth's (chapter 11) worry, that she will suddenly race outside to sit in the sun and cause herself sun-damage, is a worry that she won't allow to occur. As worries go, it could be called a fine piece of creative fiction. Worries about losing one's job, lover, or kidneys, may or may not be realistic, depending upon the facts of the situation.

Am I worrying about something serious that might happen?

Kidney failure is serious. A lupus patient who has kidney problems may end up with kidney failure. This worry, then, is about a serious concern that may come true.

"I worry that my lover will get tired of my sickness and leave me." If the lover is showing evidence of wanting to end the relationship, this, too, may be a serious concern that is likely to occur.

How to stop worrying? Decide which specific worry you want to abolish first. To get into the mood of worry-zapping, it's easiest to begin with a trivial or creative fiction one. Here are some examples:

Trivial worries. When Vera reports her Great Christmas Card Worry, everyone who doesn't worry about Christmas cards knows immediately that this worry is trivial. So are worries about cleaning the house or cooking well enough for company. Usually, worries about what other people think of your lupus rash are also trivial.

Whenever trivial worries are mentioned in groups, such as lupus support groups, other group members invariably reassure the worrier, "You don't need to worry about that." "No one cares if your Christmas card arrives on time." "I don't even send Christmas cards." "Don't worry that you haven't dusted, for heaven sakes. Nobody will even notice." "I don't worry about housecleaning, and you should see my house!" "Hey, my husband says my lupus rash is cute."

Unfortunately, such reassurances never reassure worriers. In fact, the opposite usually occurs, as the worrier insists, "You don't understand," and clings even more stubbornly to the right to escalate her worry from trivial to terrible.

One way to dispel trivial worries is to exaggerate them. It's fun to work with these worries in a group. Each member identifies her silliest trivial worry, no one is allowed to reassure the worriers, and everyone can have fun exaggerating the worries.

One woman worries, whenever she thinks her house is a bit messy, that some unexpected visitor may arrive. The story the group concocted was: Your best friend rings your doorbell, you answer, she takes one look at your living room and screams, "My God, there is dust on the mantel!" She backs out, stricken, and never visits again.

The support group invents for Vera a drama in which someone's Christmas is totally ruined by the non-arrival of Vera's Christmas card.

One woman in the group said, "Every time I come to this meeting, I worry that I might forget someone's name. That worry plagues me!" As a joke, it was decided that she should invent new names for anyone whose name she'd forgotten. If the person liked the name, she would thank her; if she didn't, she'd think up a crazy name in response.

This activity of exaggerating trivial worries, or making them silly, brings a light touch to meetings in which people are often dealing with tragedy. You can do the same thing at home. Each time that you find yourself worrying, ask yourself, "Does this worry really matter in my life or is it trivia?" If the answer is "Trivia," invent a dramatic finale. If you are worried about people seeing your rash, for instance, imagine saying, "That rash? It's nothing, just a bit of leprosy," or spin out an exaggerated "Oh, eeek!" response from the other person. If you don't like to make up silly stories, say to yourself, "I love you and I think it is OK for you to make up whatever worry you choose. And you don't have to turn it into silliness."

You can use the methods described in the chapter on autonomy, such as imagining that your inner worrier is a foolish or stupid character on television. Listen briefly and then switch channels or turn off the imaginary TV. Send the inner worrier to the moon, or enjoy inventing your own villain-zapping techniques.

Sometimes your trivial worry may be masking a real worry. The worry about your rash may be masking your concern that important people in your world are reacting badly to the fact that you are chronically ill. If so, your worry is about a serious concern.

Worries that won't come true. Beth reports, "I worry that some day I might just give up and go lie in the sun." There are two possibilities: she may be inventing this worry because she is depressed and self-destructive, or she may simply be expressing her longing for something she can't have. To know which is accurate, she imagines that she is lying in the shade under a tree, while nearby other people are in the sun. She tests the statement, "I am staying in the shade. I do take care of myself and will never hurt myself," to see if that statement feels true. If it does, fine. Her fiction was written out of longing, and she won't act on it. If she is not convinced that she will take good care of herself, she needs to test the opposite statement, "I will hurt myself by going into the sun, because ... , " and listen carefully to her answer.

She can take one side and then the other, until she has decided firmly, "I will not hurt myself for any reason, including the ones I just thought of." If she remains ambivalent about keeping herself alive, or caring for herself well, she needs to find a good therapist who can work with her on overcoming depression, and on issues of self-care versus self-abuse.

When she is certain that she will not hurt herself, she can tell herself kindly, whenever she has her fantasy about going out into the sunshine, "It's all right to imagine being in the sun. Fantasy and reality are different. I can fantasy whatever I like because I won't do anything to hurt myself." By telling herself this, she is affirming the difference between thoughts and actions, and re-enforcing her willingness to care for herself. She's also learning another way to deal with worry, by simply saying, "Of course I won't do that," or "Of course that won't happen."

She may turn her worry into silliness. For example, she imagines headlines in the local newspaper: "Woman Attempts Suicide By Lying In Sun! Saved By Neighborhood Kindergartner Who Drags Her Into Shade And Hoses Her Off."

One woman worries that she will run out of money for her care, even though this is impossible in her circumstances. She exaggerates her story about future poverty and lack of care until the story totally bores her. Each time she gives herself a worry that won't come true, she does the same thing, exaggerating it to the point of boredom.

Worries about serious concerns that might come true. Remember, worrying never helps, so you'll want to banish these worries, too. But first, ask yourself, "What can I do to try to prevent this worry from coming true?" Worrying won't get you a cold beer on a hot day, but planning and carrying out plans may help avoid the outcomes you fear.

Worrying doesn't save kidneys, and even with the best diet, fluid intake, exercise, and medical attention, if your kidneys are affected by your lupus, they may fail. It's still worthwhile to do everything you can to prolong their life.

If a person worries that a relationship is not working out, the person may tell her lover her concerns and desires, listen to the lover's responses, and attempt to make their life together happy, but no one has power over others. We cannot change the way others feel, think, or behave. We are only in charge of ourselves.

A young woman with lupus said, "Now that I have The Rash and I'm fat because of steroids, no one will want to marry me." Lots of lupus sufferers worry that they won't find a love partner. That is a serious concern that might come true, although Pamela's and Mitch's (chapter 3) romance began in the hospital when she was seriously ill with lupus, and Tamara doesn't seem to have difficulties finding menfriends.

How do you find a person who will love you, lupus and all? Instead of worrying that you'll never be loved, learn to love yourself. When you love yourself, you know in your heart that you don't have to have a partner in order to be happy. You know that you alone are in charge of your own happiness. You are searching for a partner who will share your happiness rather than bring you happiness. When you love yourself and create your own happiness, you can't help demonstrating your happiness and inner security wherever you are, in grocery stores, doctor's offices, or at work. People who enjoy happy partners will notice you. Also, when you already know how to be happy, your search for a partner can be fun rather than desperate.

To find a partner, then, the first step is to recognize your own worth. The next step is to look for someone as interesting and lovable and special as you. You do need a plan for meeting such a person.

Sleeping Beauty is a fiction. There aren't worthwhile princes who are searching arduously for princesses who are lying comatose in their own attics.

Figure out where to go and what to do to meet people who would make good partners. To find men, go to the places where there are lots of them. Peek into adult classrooms, and enroll in the classes where most of the students are males in your age group. Try launderettes, chess tournaments, ball games, and political clubs. By the same token, men can find women where they congregate: in the classroom, churches, clubs, and places of work. If you are lesbian, go where there are women who love women, in special clubs, organizations, church groups, or bars. Everyone looking for a partner or a friend ought to check with the chamber of commerce for lists of clubs and interest groups in the area, and pick the ones that appeal.

Here is a sampling of places where you are sure to find nice people: craft shops, symphonies, museums, and art shows. When you see someone who is alone, say, "Oh, do you like that painting? I do."

Rialta (chapter 4) worries that she'll have a bowel obstruction and end up with a colostomy. "I have an irregular bowel and a partial obstruction. Some physicians say this is not a symptom of lupus and others say that it is. I worry because the doctors are not definite." On top of this worry she adds a fictional worry, "I worry that if I think about it, it will come true."

Lots of people act as if thinking about something will make it so. That is the ostrich approach to life, hiding one's head in the sand in order to feel safe. It's a dangerous stance for lupus patients.

Rialta needs to find out what, if anything, she can do to cure a partial obstruction and to prevent further obstruction. What diet is best and what research is being reported? For everyone, getting information is a positive approach, while worrying is not. Instead of worrying, she can read, ask questions, and scan the internet. If she doesn't know how to use the internet, Dr. Fagan's (Appendix) article will tell her exactly how to do it.

Sometimes worrying is an indication that the person is still reacting to past traumas. Traumas are events in people's lives that are more than they can handle emotionally, and therefore may continue to cause nervousness and worry. If you've once been struck by lightning, it's difficult to contemplate an electrical storm without worrying.

For lupus patients, worries about future catastrophes such as kidney failure, poverty, or death may be in part a reaction to past, unresolved traumatic experiences. Everyone who suffers from lupus has experienced trauma. For you it may have been sudden, intense pain, a frightening hospitalization, near strangulation such as Louise (chapter 10) survived, or a sudden loss of memory. People tend to discount the effects of trauma on their lives. They don't know why they are chronically worried, because no one has suggested to them that worrying may be a signal that a past trauma needs to be dealt with.

It takes time and sometimes skilled help to recover from trauma. There are several ways of dealing with memories of past trauma. The easiest is to tell yourself in detail and as simply as possible, what happened to you. Listen to yourself and say aloud, "That was terrible," "I have a right to feel distress and pain about that," "I am sorry I suffered so much." Make up your own loving, caring words to yourself.

Let yourself feel and express your feelings. It is important to sob, be furious, and to feel very, very sorry for yourself. Know that recovery is especially difficult for people who suppress their emotions. As you keep your recital simple, and give yourself only loving responses, you are healing yourself as you talk.

You are a unique person, and what was traumatic for you may not be traumatic for others. For you, being naked in an emergency room when your gown slips to one side may be more traumatic than the pain you were suffering. Let yourself mourn your feelings of loss of dignity, loss of pride, and loss of control. Any of these may have been unbearable for you. Know and accept your own past pains and humiliations without judging them.

You also need help from others. Pick a friend, relative, or pastor who will listen lovingly, and tell that person what happened to you. An empathic listener follows these rules: don't give advice, don't change the subject, don't talk about someone else with the same or worse problem. Give understanding.

A support group is invaluable because it is easier to speak about your hurts to those who have suffered similarly.

When you have learned to unblock your feelings, comfort yourself, and accept comfort from others, you are ready to say good-bye to the past. Remember the traumatic scene in detail, allow yourself to express your feelings in that scene, and then when you are ready, say "Good-bye." Afterwards, you may still think about your trauma from time to time, but you will be more free to separate your present from your past. Once you have resolved old traumas, you won't spend as much energy worrying about ones that have not yet occurred.

If you continue to be burdened by childhood traumas, or you aren't recovering from the traumas in your adult life, find a good psychotherapist. It might be the best gift you have ever given yourself.

After doing whatever you can to prevent serious concerns from becoming reality, it is time to let those worries go. Trade worrying for serenity by practicing breathing exercises or imagining a lovely trip on your magic carpet over fields of waving, many-colored flowers.

For hard-core worriers, or anyone who doesn't like fantasy trips, behavior modification approaches are also helpful. Buy yourself a stroke counter (for counting golf strokes) in a sporting goods store and wear it all the time. Whenever you begin to worry, no matter what the content of the worry, simply click the starter. At the end of each day, write down or chart the number of clicks for that day. The number of worries per day will begin to decline after a few days or weeks. Another option is to worry only on schedule. Decide for yourself exactly when and where you will worry and how much time you will spend worrying. Three minutes, twice a day? Before each meal? Only when you are showering? Dressing? Doing dishes? Any time is all right, and any place except in your bed. Beds are sacred and must not be used for worrying, arguing, or any other negative activity. Beds are for love and rest.

After you have decided when and where to worry, make certain that you keep to the schedule. If you start to worry at a non-designated time, remind yourself, "I'll worry about this during my worry period but not now."

You have sorted through your worries and done what you can do to take good care of yourself and your loved ones, and you have learned lots of techniques for ridding yourself of worrying.

Along the way, you must have noticed that you can't really do much about preventing some worries from coming true. No matter how much you worry about other people, you can't make them do what you want. You may not be able to prevent sick kidneys from ceasing to function. You can't cure your lupus. You can't keep anyone from dying some day. In fact, you can't get guarantees about the future.

Think of your worries as heavy stones that you have been dragging around with you. Each stone represents a problem that might some day be reality, but is not your reality now. Imagine the weight of this bag of stones on your shoulders and back, which are already tired and pained from lupus.

Put down your bag of heavy stones, open it, and take out one stone at a time. Imagine that beside the bag of stones is a deep hole. Identify each stone as one of your old worries, say to the stone, "I am not carrying you any longer," and drop it into the hole. When you have finished with all the stones, toss the sack in after them.

When the going gets tough, instead of worrying, you may want to say aloud the Serenity Prayer:

God grant me the strength to accept the things I cannot change, courage to change the things I can, and the wisdom to know the difference.

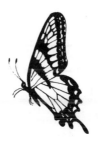

28

Be Assertive For Your Health's Sake

Remember Joyce (chapter 8) in the hospital emergency room, insisting to the doctor, "I have a perforated colon." She refused to allow him to order lab tests that would waste time or be harmful to her in her critical condition. She established her credentials, "I've been through this before. I know what is going on inside me." When he didn't believe her, she said, "You are going to listen to me!" and told him to call her own physician. "I am in a lot of pain, so hurry." Later, her physician said that her assertiveness saved her life.

Assertiveness is the ability to know your own desires or needs, and to communicate them potently and effectively. That is exactly what Joyce did. Hers was an emergency situation, in which she did a spectacular job of getting her needs known to the physician.

Assertiveness helps both the giver and the receiver of the message. When an assertive statement seems to be hurtful to another person, probably it was aggressive rather than assertive. The aggressor tramples on the rights of another person, hurting, belittling, manipulating, or overpowering her. Aggressive behavior comes from a win-lose philosophy, which suggests that for every victory someone must be victimized.

Assertiveness doesn't mean winning at someone else's expense; in fact, the concept of win-lose is inappropriate, because assertiveness is based on respect for oneself and respect for others. Joyce wasn't asserting herself in order to prove that she was in some way superior to the emergency room doctor. In this critical situation, she was insisting that her body get needed care quickly. Her insistence was life-saving for her and important to the doctor as well. Every physician wants to save lives and, without her help, he might have failed.

Assertiveness is not only for emergency use. Beth (chapter 11) understood the day-by-day value of assertiveness. She said, "I have explained to everyone at work exactly what is wrong with me. I don't deny my pain, or pretend I can do things that hurt me. For example, I discovered that the halogen light over my desk was giving me trouble, so I asked that it be replaced with a different kind of lighting." Her assertiveness at work minimizes misunderstandings, and helps her to be able to continue working in spite of lupus.

When we know what we want and communicate it, our lives become richer, easier, and more intimate. Just the simple communication of where to go to dinner is enhanced by the willingness of each person to be assertive. "I would like Italian food. What appeals to you?" It is frustrating when the other person's usual response is, "I don't know," "I don't care," or, "Whatever you say."

For a lupus patient, a first step in learning to be assertive is to know what is best for her. Does a certain prescribed drug help? Some people are very much helped by drugs that others find completely useless or, worse, harmful. You may do well with an anti-depressant or a tranquilizer that your friends in the lupus support group swear is ineffective. You may end up groggy and unable to function if you take a sleeping pill that gives others a much-needed night of rest. If you don't pay attention to your own feelings of comfort and discomfort, or don't reveal what you know, you won't be giving accurate information to your doctor. The non-responsive, "Anything you say," may merely label you boring or frustrating when the subject is restaurants. "Anything you say," when said by a lupus patient to her doctor about her own body, is extremely dangerous.

As Dr. Press (chapter 21) stated, "From my perspective, the most important attribute for health is self-care. What does self-care mean? It means that the individual is responsive and responsible, rather than passive, in the treatment of her illness."

Another important aspect of assertiveness is the recognition of one's own personal boundaries. Each individual is unique, and has the right to have her physical and psychological boundaries respected. Are you comfortable when people stand very close to you, talk loudly in your face, put an arm around you without asking your permission, call you by your first name rather than ask how you would like to be addressed? Each of these actions is a potential boundary violation that may happen to you, unless you tell others your preferences. "I prefer to be called Ms. Jones." "I know you are being friendly, but I want you to ask my permission before you hug me." "Please stand back a bit. I feel overpowered when anyone stands too close." "Please talk a bit more softly. I'll still hear you. Thank you."

Your psychological boundaries are violated when you are told, rather than asked, what you feel or think. "You don't want to go outside today, honey. It's chilly." Or, "This doesn't really hurt." Many health-care workers ignore patients' boundaries by misuse of the word "we," as in, "We are going to be brave, aren't we?" or the classic, "Now it is time for our enema." Everyone has a right to claim her own thoughts and feelings, and enemas.

Sometimes lupus patients avoid being assertive by using what is called "catastrophizing." They believe, "If I ask for what I want, something terrible will happen." When invited to imagine, "What is the worst thing that could happen," they say, "My doctor may give up on me," or "My son will be angry," or "My partner may leave me." In this way, even if they know what they need or want, and know how to express themselves well, their expectations of rejection get in their way. They substitute worry for action.

Some of these worries are totally unreal, and others are based on what has happened in the past. If you are dealing with an angry or controling person, he or she may misinterpret your assertiveness for aggression, and respond angrily. Such people often don't listen well, because they fear losing command of any situation. You may have to invite them to express their concerns first, reassure them, and then gently maintain your own assertive position.

If you are assertive with an abusive person, you may risk being abused. If you are assertive with an undependable person, that person may agree with your stance and then let you down. In these situations, the problem is not your assertiveness, but your relationship with people who are not willing to respect your feelings and needs.

When Beth (chapter 11) returned to the rheumatologist who told her she didn't have lupus, he responded sarcastically, "Sure, now that you know what the symptoms are, you've managed to develop the right symptoms." Beth was humiliated. She was also "angry enough to choose a different rheumatologist," which she did. Tamara (chapter 13) ended her seven-year relationship with a lover who was unwilling to respond positively when she told him her needs. Assertiveness is not a magic potion. It is a way to communicate well with people who are worthy of your respect and friendship. Perhaps another advantage of assertiveness is that your assertiveness can help you decide who will remain important in your life.

If you have difficulty asserting yourself, the problem may be based on your childhood experiences. Dolores (chapter 6) seemed to accept the tragic beliefs: "There's nothing I can do" and "No one will listen to me, anyway." She expected no one to help her, because that had been her experience since childhood. "When I was a child, I had pains. I used to curl up in a ball, I had so much pain all over. My mother didn't believe me. She thought I was making it all up, so that I wouldn't have to go to school, but I wasn't. I quit school in the sixth grade because of my pain." No one dealt effectively with her pain in childhood, and no one is dealing effectively with her lupus today.

One reason she is now very ill is that she does not demand good care. She says, "I wish they'd give me something for the lupus, something that would make me better, but I haven't got a lupus doctor. Lupus doctors don't come to this nursing home." She is a Medicaid patient, who seems to go along with the belief of many taxpayers, that the poor deserve only second-rate care. Of course, society pays much more to keep her drugged in a nursing home than they would pay if she were seen by a physician who treated her lupus so that she could recover from flares, get off morphine, and live in her own home with her friend.

Many women have adapted to social messages that keep them from being assertive. "Women shouldn't be pushy," "It's a woman's job to keep the peace," or "Men (including male doctors) don't like women who act too smart." Are you willing to oppose such chauvinistic slogans?

Change "Women shouldn't be pushy," to "I will not be a pushover." "It's a woman's job to keep the peace," can become, "Peace comes from respecting and being respected." Change "Men don't like smart women" to "Truly intelligent men appreciate intelligent women."

There are lots of beliefs that keep patients from asserting themselves. Another is the fear that a doctor will find that they aren't "really sick." Patients believe that, unless the doctor discovers that the patient is "really sick," the doctor will think she has wasted her time. When a problem is diagnosed as minor, such patients actually feel ashamed rather than relieved. They would almost rather hear, "You are so sick that you need to be hospitalized immediately," because then no one can accuse them of lying about their symptoms. Any doctor will tell you that it is a cause for rejoicing, for doctor and patient, whenever a medical problem is not serious!

If you have difficulty asserting yourself, you may be blocked by beliefs about yourself, which you project onto others, such as "they'll think I'm selfish," "self-centered," "a complainer," "whiner," "weak," "unable to take a little pain," "a hypochondriac." The saddest beliefs of all are "I'm not lovable," and "I'm not important."

Make a list of the negative beliefs that you have used to hold yourself back, so that you can get rid of them.

You might want to show your list to other members of your lupus support group. An interesting activity at support group meetings is for each person to make a list of negative beliefs that keep her from being assertive, and read them aloud. Group members listen, share, and invent silly responses to each item. They help each other substitute positive beliefs that encourage assertiveness, and then burn their old lists.

If you are working alone on your list, bring in all the helpful selves inside your head. That way you can have your very own group. Include your personal fairy godmother, pals, admirers, and the loving people from your past and present that you put into your head in exchange for your villains. Show them your list and let them change your self-negating messages into affirmations. Be sure to start with, "I am important."

When you believe that you are important, unique, and deserving of attention from others, you are ready to learn assertive techniques.

Think of a situation in which you want to express a desire or need. Meg (chapter 12) reported that when her laboratory tests were negative, the doctor tried to slough her off, saying that maybe she simply needed to rest more. She told him, "No matter what the tests say, there is something very wrong in my body, and I want you to find out what it is." Her doctor then decided to test for lupus, even though he had never heard of anyone getting lupus after menopause. It turned out that at age fifty-eight she had lupus.

Perhaps you want to tell your doctor, "I took my name off the list for a kidney transplant because I wasn't ready to face the surgery, and now I am ready. Please put me back on the list," or "I have decided that I want to consult a rheumatologist, in order to have a second opinion on my lupus. Whom do you recommend?"

Perhaps you want to tell your daughter, "Tonight I need to go to bed early. I don't want dishes left in the sink, because of the problem we've been having with ants in the kitchen. Before you go to bed, please put the dishes in the dishwasher and clean off the counters. Another day, when I am feeling better, I'll do the clean-up."

You might want to tell your partner, "I promised that I'd go with you to the Elks' picnic, and that was a mistake. I don't feel well, and I know being in the sun will make me worse. I have decided not to go." Notice that in each example, the message is specific.

Here are examples of non-assertive statements to be avoided:

"My neighbor once saw a specialist. Do lots of people see specialists?" or, to your daughter, "I want you to help me more in the kitchen," or to your partner, "I think maybe I should try to stay out of the sun more often." You cannot be assertive by talking in generalities. Say exactly what you want.

"If you wouldn't mind too much ..." This is weak, ineffective, and gives away your right to choose for yourself.

"Up to now I've tried to do everything you want, but this once ..." This is the sort of martyred statement that will get you sighs, plus arguments about what you have and haven't done.

"I need a doctor who knows what's wrong with me!" Or, "You never help around the house!" These statements are insulting and aggressive rather than assertive.

After telling the other person clearly what you want or need, the next step is to listen intelligently to the response you receive. Sometimes, if you listen carefully, you'll hear an even better solution than the one you presented. Your physician may suggest a nephrologist, because he is concerned about your kidneys. Your daughter may ask that in the future paper plates be used when neither of you wants kitchen duties. Your partner may suggest that you arrive at the picnic at sundown, in time for the evening festivities. Compromises leave each person feeling understood and important.

If the other person asks for more information, give it freely. "It's not just sun. Heat and dust bother me. And when my body aches this much, it isn't fun to go to a place where everyone else is partying." "The reason I'm not willing to clean the kitchen is that I'm in the middle of another flare. Yesterday I started taking Prednisone again, and in a couple of days I should be a lot better."

Sometimes, the other person proposes distractions, procrastination, or arguments. If the doctor says, "Yes, well, we'll talk about that another time," you can say, "I know you are busy, and I do want the name of a rheumatologist today."

Answer, if possible, by agreeing with what is said, and then repeat your own statement. "Of course, this picnic is important to you and you have a right to resent my being sick so often, and I am glad that you give me your honest response. Even so, I am not going to the picnic."

"Yes, I know your favorite TV show is tonight. I hope you can watch it and finish your homework. Whether you can do it all or not, please put the dishes in the dishwasher and clean off the counters before you go to bed."

If the other person is critical of you, it is usually best to agree, while you continue to be firm about what you want. "Yes, that's true, I should have decided to have the kidney transplant when one was available. That was stupid of me, and now I do want to be back on the list." "Yes, you have a right to complain when I change my mind at the last moment, and I am not going."

You may need to be persistent, if the other person isn't used to hearing you stick up for yourself, or if the situation causes problems for the other person.

Sometimes, there doesn't seem to be a way to arrive at a solution. Either of you may become angry, stubborn, hurt, and unwilling to compromise. In such situations, suggest a "time out" and a return to the discussion at a later, specified time.

Are you ready to practice assertiveness? Choose a specific problem and solution you want to communicate to an employer or employee, friend, physician, health-care worker, or family member. In teaching yourself to be assertive, it's easier to begin with a situation in which the other person is likely to agree with you. Postpone the tough issues until you feel competent.

When you've picked your situation, imagine the scene in which you and the other person are together. Silently, remind yourself that you are important and lovable, and then tell the person what you want or need, and explain clearly your reasons for your statements. Be factual and pleasant, rather than argumentative or timid. If you believe that the other person will try to sidetrack you, practice acknowledging what he or she said, and then repeating your assertive statement. Continue the imaginary dialogue until you are satisfied with your part in it, and then critique yourself.

Were you clear, concise, and kind? Did you stay on track? Practice the scene several times, if you like, until you are satisfied with your ability to be assertive. The final step is to do the scene in reality, as soon as possible after you have practiced it in your imagination.

If the real-life scene doesn't turn out as you expected it would, practice again by using a different scene and different person. If you still are having difficulties, read books on assertiveness training or see a counselor, who could point out your blind spots.

When your real-life scene turns out in a way that satisfies you, be sure to give genuine appreciation to whoever was the recipient of your assertiveness. "Dr. Jones, I was worried about discussing this with you, and I want you to know how appreciative I am of your willingness to hear me out. Thank you very much." To your partner, you might send a rose with the note, "Thanks for your understanding. I love you." To your daughter or son, give a hug, a statement of appreciation, and occasionally a small thank-you present.

Assertiveness is a two-way street. Everyone wants to feel respected and heard, so encourage people in your life to be assertive with you. When you establish a win-win philosophy in your relationships with others, your life and theirs will be richer for it.

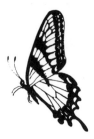

29

Your Work Life
And What To Do If You Can't Work

Most important of all: don't quit your job when you first become ill! No matter how sick you are, do whatever you can to keep your job. The chances are excellent that you will be less sick soon. As Dr. Barber said, "Lupus is a disease that can be identified, understood, possibly controlled; and the progression of the disease can be slowed down." In the beginning, you may be so sick that the idea of never working again is appealing, but once you start to feel better, you might well change your mind. Give yourself a chance to be stabilized before making any long-term changes in your life.

Even if at first you are very ill, unable to move or in incredible pain, don't give up your employment. Take sick leave, vacation leave, leave without pay, but wait to decide about your future employment until your lupus is under better control, and you and your doctor can make an intelligent assessment of your condition. Dr. Barber encourages patients "to continue with whatever makes their lives worthwhile, not to withdraw from life, and to keep moving beyond the limitations their disease may seem to impose." Remember, for chronically ill people it is easier to keep a job than to find a new one.

If you are too confused or depressed to care about the future, ask someone to be your advocate. That person, a friend or relative, can deal with insurance companies and your employers, so that you don't precipitously lose out, as Vera did when she ran from her job. Your advocate will help you until you can do your own planning.

After your medication has begun to be effective, and you start feeling better, you may be faced with the big question, "To work or not to work."

Tamara said, "I was constantly worried that I might have to stop working. I suppose that is a worry facing all lupus patients who like or need their jobs. I had purchased disability insurance before I had lupus, so I could manage financially if I decided to quit working, but my self-esteem was involved. It was vitally important to me that I earn my own money and be independent. To me, to be unemployable would be far more punishing than to be in pain. I love my work."

If you, like Tamara, want to work, you'll need to assess very carefully whether you can continue with your type of employment, and what compromises might be necessary in order to keep working. Explain your physical difficulties and limitations to your employer, and ask your employer to accommodate to your limitations or disabilities. You cannot be fired simply because you are disabled. Employers are mandated to make needed changes in your work place so that you can remain employed.

If you can't walk, request a desk job at least temporarily. If you can no longer lift heavy objects, you may have to stop floor nursing, for example, but you can be reassigned to audit charts or do discharge planning. If you are in the police force, you can be given a desk assignment.

Find furniture that is comfortable at work. If you can't sit through a normal day of work, get permission to take a fifteen-minute nap when you need one.

Experiment with what you can and can't do. Make your work life as easy as possible by looking for ways to avoid both physical and emotional stress at work.

Explain your lupus symptoms to your colleagues. Help them understand that every lupus sufferer is different. Your symptoms, like your capabilities, are unique. Some of your colleagues may have friends with lupus who are healthier than you, and others may know people who are incapacitated by the disease. That's why it's important for you to let them know your own unique problems. Make friends with the colleagues who are supportive.

Tamara said, "I don't deny my pain, or pretend I can do things that hurt me. I keep careful track of what is going on inside my body, and try to figure out accurately what causes my flares. For example, I discovered that the halogen light over my desk was giving me trouble, so I asked that it be replaced with a different kind of lighting."

She found that she could only commute to work two consecutive days without a rest, so on Wednesdays she works out of her own home. She explained, "Everyone understands my need for an easy schedule, and makes allowances when I sometimes have to take a quick nap in the middle of the day."

Working at home is a good alternative for anyone like Tamara, whose employment includes a fair amount of time on the computer. If you are interested in doing your work part-time or full-time at home, figure out how you can do this. Take out a pen and paper and let your imagination run wild. Don't censor or argue against any of your ideas. You are looking for creative ways of continuing the job you have. What search could be more important? Test your new ideas to see if some of them can meet your desires and your employer's needs.

If you decide that you cannot remain in the old job, look for potential new jobs, but don't rush to quit your old employment. A good idea would be to talk with an employment consultant, who knows about jobs that can be done at home. You may need to study for a totally new career. One of the women in a lupus support group has become a travel agent, because her previous job was too taxing. She can imagine taking each trip that she plans for her clients, and she specializes in trips for the disabled.

IF YOU CANNOT CONTINUE TO WORK

When you can't continue to work, you will want to apply

for state disability; COBRA, the federally mandated program for medical insurance; Social Security; and any private disability insurance you have.

Get ready to apply for all of them before you quit your job. How to get ready? First, explain to the physician who knows your medical problems, why you and/or your employer believe that you can't continue to work. A diagnosis of SLE is not sufficient by itself to allow you to be on state disability or Social Security.

Objective evidence of inability to work, such as kidney failure and the need for dialysis, will always be accepted as evidence that you cannot continue your employment. If you don't have such objective evidence, remind your doctor of the subjective evidence that you cannot work, such as inability to concentrate, forgetfulness, memory loss, pain, fatigue, chronic nausea or diarrhea, etc. Report any disabilities that disqualify you from continuing in your present employment: inability to type, if you are a secretary; inability to lift heavy objects, if you work for a moving company; or inability to stand for long periods of time, if you are a checker in a supermarket. Make a list of what is required of you at work, and which of these tasks are beyond your current ability. Make certain that your physician puts down in your medical record both subjective and objective disabilities, and ask for a copy of the medical record. If you have seen more than one physician, you'll need to get copies of their records, too.

It's best to go on sick leave while applying for benefits, because if your claims are denied, it may become impossible for you to find another job.

File for state disability. Each state has slightly different requirements. You can find out about your state disability regulations by calling the department of employment in your state. In California you must fill out a single form, which is almost always accepted on a physician's recommendation. The maximum payment in California is $336 a week, payable every other week. It takes effect two weeks after you have stopped working. You can collect it only for one year. You may begin collecting state disability even if you are still on the payroll, using your sick leave or vacation pay, for example.

Keep your medical insurance. You will need to buy your own medical insurance, using COBRA, the federally mandated program that allows you to continue the same health insurance you had while working. Supposedly you'll be charged only two percent above cost; however, expect the cost to shoot up. If the medical benefit plan cost $250 while you were working, it may cost $350 a month when you have to pay it yourself under COBRA. You can keep this insurance for a maximum of eighteen months. Make sure that you pay insurance premiums on time every month, or your insurance can be cut off.

Apply for Supplementary Security Income. If your only assets are your home, car, and no more than $2000 in other assets, you qualify for Supplementary Security Income, or SSI. You will receive a maximum of only $660 a month, but, in addition, SSI pays your medical expenses, which can run into thousands of dollars. Meg, on SSI, cannot afford to accept her potentially excellent social security, because on social security a person has to pay her own medical bills for two years. Even when she is not hospitalized, Meg's bills are more than $1000 every month. As Meg reported, it is not easy to live on $660 a month, but people on SSI in many areas do receive free housing. If you are poor and have high medical expenses, SSI may be your best bet.

Social Security. Disability under Social Security is awarded when the Social Security Administration agrees that you are unable to work because of your disability. You will be considered disabled if you are unable to do work for which you are suited, and your disability is expected to last for at least a year, or to result in death.

If you qualify for social security benefits, you will receive whatever is due you, depending on your salary and years of employment, regardless of the assets you possess. Your spouse and children also qualify for benefits when you are on social security for your disability. You can find out what you and your family would receive, by telephoning the social security 800 number or going to a social security office in your area.

When you apply for social security, you need to fill out the various forms they will give you, and take them, with copies of your medical records, to your social security office. Keep copies of every form you fill out, plus copies of all of your medical records! You will be sent to additional physicians chosen by the social security administration, and will be required to fill out at least two more sets of forms. You need the originals of all paper work, including those filled out by your physician, in order to fill out correctly the additional paper work. It is a big job, especially if you are suffering and incapacitated.

It is your responsibility to see to it that these files are accurate. Remember to answer all questions as briefly as possible, in accordance with what is in your physician's files. If you are not physically or emotionally able to do all of this, you can hire specialists who will do the job for you. The social security office has lists of specialists. You can also, of course, find family or friends who are able to handle the paper work for you.

After you have kept all your appointments and turned in all your paper work, the Social Security office will review your application and send it to the Disability Determination Services office (DDS) in your state. There, in about three - five months, a determination will be made, and you will receive a written notice of the decision. If you are approved, you will receive your first disability check, which will include payments dating back to the sixth full month from the date when your disability began. If you are not approved, you need to appeal immediately. At this point, you may decide to hire someone to assist you in presenting your claim.

Once you have been approved for social security, all other public and private plans will agree that you are disabled. That is the good news. The bad news: even after you begin receiving social security, you are still responsible for your own medical bills. You don't qualify for Medicare until you have been on social security for two years. This is, of course, crazy. If you cannot work because you are chronically ill, you are obviously in need of medical care, and have no means of working to provide for your care. Nevertheless, this is the law. And this is why Meg is on SSI rather than Social Security, to which she is entitled.

To manage your medical care for those two years, keep your COBRA medical benefits for the full eighteen months, and then find some other way to pay your medical bills for the six months until you qualify for medicare.

Private disability insurance. Hopefully, you have privately-financed disability insurance that you have purchased or was purchased for you through your company or union. These usually pay sixty percent of your salary when you cannot work because of a disability. All working people ought to carry private insurance, but many healthy people choose to ignore the fact that they could become chronically ill. If you were foresighted enough to get private insurance, you probably can retire comfortably, using the insurance plus social security. Check to be sure you are also receiving your share of any pension plans that you, your spouse, or ex-spouse may have.

When you have stopped working, your task is to keep your life interesting. At first, especially if you are quite ill, television may be a good distraction, but look for more than that. Take correspondence courses; do volunteer work for your favorite charity, perhaps the Lupus Foundation of America; start a lupus support group in your neighborhood; tend your garden after sundown; make yourself an exercise schedule; visit friends. You might decide to raise and sell aquarium fish, or acquire a well-behaved pet to keep you company. Your number-one priority is to make your retirement enjoyable and stimulating.

Meg discovered that she was eligible for free tickets to musical events and museums, as well as for scholarships for college courses. She pickets for the rights of the handicapped. Vera is a leader of a group that raises money for disabled children. Joyce and Maria make beautiful handicrafts. One benefit of joining a lupus support group is that you will hear how other women are managing to have happy lives.

Discover for yourself that retirement can be an adventure.

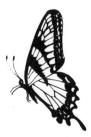

30

Your Home Life
How To Make It Richer, Easier and More Fun

For everyone, happiness at home makes all the difference. No matter what symptoms you have, a good home-life enhances your mental and physical health. An unhappy, stressful home-life may injure both your psyche and your body. As Tamara said, when she decided to separate from Patrick, "He was not good for me emotionally or financially ... I had more flares and was using more steroids with fewer positive results. The pain in my joints was increasing." After leaving Patrick, she found a "kind, generous, low-keyed man who likes to go out once in a while but is also content at home with me. I am healthier, I think, but the important part is that I am happy and therefore don't agitate myself about my health."

Partners. All partners have disagreements. Some are quietly rational in their struggles, and some scream and shout. Style doesn't matter, as long as they resolve issues and enjoy each other. At this point in your life, as you feel ugly from weight gain and rashes, have little energy, are depressed and in pain, you are apt to be very vulnerable to even the tiniest slights or disagreements. Your partner is also vulnerable, perhaps because he feels helpless and frightened. He may feel trapped and resentful but doesn't dare say so. Lupus is a crisis that affects both the patient and those dearest to her, and can either cement a marriage or destroy it. If you have worries about you and your partner, find a competent couples' therapist to help you through the trauma of your illness. You don't need to consider yourself a "mental case" to get help. If you have relatives who would like to help you financially, this is a fine way to use their money.

189

With or without therapy, couples need to show each other love, and be supportive. When two people are successful in this, their attachment almost invariably deepens.

Joyce's problems were unusually severe. "Within two months of our honeymoon I was temporarily a quadriplegic. Art, my new husband, had to dress me, brush my teeth, do everything for me. I couldn't even open my own mouth." Their love for each other carried them through these terrible months.

Stan, Maria's husband, believes, "Her lupus made us stronger." Maria agrees with him. She says, "Stan is my best friend." Like Stan and Maria and Joyce and Art, you and your partner may discover increased intimacy from sharing feelings about your disease, working together at home, and comforting each other.

Children. Children whose mothers have lupus are like all children, a product of their environment and their own genetic predisposition. Some are easy to live with and some are difficult, depending upon how their innate personalities fit into the family and blend with the personalities of others.

In addition to normal childhood problems, your children have to live with the stress of your illness. This stress is harder on some children than others. Just as some children react very well to the entrance of another child into the family and some don't, some children react well to a mother's illness and some are negatively affected by it. Those who are naturally calm may be easier for you to cope with than those who are hyperactive, restless, or irritable.

Neither you nor your child created your child's intrinsic personality, or your current problems. You are not responsible for your lupus, and your child is not responsible for the genetic structure that he or she inherited. Blaming children for their response to your illness is inappropriate as well as ineffective.

Some quick do's and don'ts. Don't overburden a helpful child. Get relief from a difficult child by hiring sitters or bringing in relatives and friends to help you. Your best bet is to find an adolescent or an adult who likes your child. It is cause for joy, not shame, when someone else seems to handle your child more easily than you do.

Give hugs, kisses, and lots of verbal praise whenever a child does something positive, and ignore as much of the negative behavior as you can. Love your child, show your love, and spend much more time praising happiness than analyzing unhappiness.

The fewer the rules, the easier your life will be. Only you can decide what behavior is unacceptable, and remember that pointing out the unacceptable lets a rebellious child know exactly how to push your buttons.

If your child seems unusually sad, anxious, or angry in reaction to your illness, ask yourself if you are modelling happy behavior. Of course, you don't want to paste a false smile on your face. Children are sensitive to both body language and words, so if the two are incongruous, the kids will sense this, and be doubly anxious as they try to sort out the lies from the truth.

With children, it is best to be as truthful as possible. You may need to reassure your child that you are not dying and that you expect to feel better soon. Explain that lupus is a strange disease that causes an adult to feel terrible one day and just fine the next. This is very understandable to children, whose earaches or stomach upsets seem to come and go. Promise to tell your child if your sickness gets worse, and keep that promise.

Don't let anyone, family, partner, or friends, blame your child for your illness, or suggest that a child's behavior can make you feel better or worse. The guilt induced by such statements lasts a lifetime.

Trying to be your child's therapist will drive you both nutty. If your child needs professional help, find a family therapist for all of you.

For your sake as well as your child's sake, look for happy moments to share. Make time to draw pictures together. Enjoy with your child the sight of a beautiful bird, the sound of bells, the soft feeling of hugging together. Tell your child, "I love the way you smile." Read aloud humorous children's books.

Housework. Your home may be a house or apartment, a quiet, private, very personal sanctuary, or a bustling gathering place for the whole neighborhood. It may be plain or fancy. No matter what kind of home you have, it requires upkeep that may be beyond your ability and strength, especially during the early stages of your lupus.

Without help, the stress of overdoing and never quite catching up can deplete your energy and even destroy your love for your own home. Before that happens to you, you need to figure out ways of getting the household jobs done.

Set priorities. Decide which jobs need to be done and which jobs you merely want done, and know the difference. Needs are essential for life and health. Wants are just about everything else. Write down the essential tasks, such as providing food, taking out garbage, laundering. When you can't do these jobs, they must be assigned to others.

Important though non-vital tasks, such as watering a lawn and cleaning your house, come next on your list. Again, you may ask others to help you or, when you have an interlude of good health, you can do them yourself. The not-that-important tasks on your list, such as washing windows or raising a vegetable garden, can be postponed until you feel well enough to handle them.

Nikki lost her garden during those first months of her illness, and now, like many lupus patients, she has the strength and energy to create a new garden. In setting priorities, remind yourself that you will feel better in the future. Lots of household tasks can wait.

If you are attempting to continue working in your job or profession in spite of your lupus, your health is still your first priority. If possible, use some of the money you earn to hire help for housework. If you think you can't afford help, then look at your spending priorities. People live quite well without expensive food, and hired help is much more important than new clothes.

Find short cuts. When you feel well enough to cook, fix a lot of food and freeze leftovers for the days when you are not up to cooking. Substitute carry-out food for home-cooked meals. Rest before dinner, even if that means the dinner will be late. Accept offers for meals brought to your home.

More suggestions: If you are guilty about a letter you haven't sent, make a phone call instead. Never use a scrub brush; use a mop. If you are too tired to put away the laundry, don't hassle yourself. Eventually, you'll move the clothes from the pile on the dining room table to their proper places. Don't iron clothes. Anything that must be ironed can be given to Goodwill. Ask a friend to do your grocery shopping at the same time that she does her own. Choose a friend who likes cleaning and is a whiz at it, and ask if she would help you clean your house once a month.

In the past, you may have kept an immaculate home; that is no longer realistic. Perhaps you loved to re-paint your walls almost every year, and to make new drapes and pillows. Until you are much healthier, you need to be satisfied with the paint that is already on your walls.

If you live alone, your house or apartment will never get as dirty as the homes of friends with partners and children. Believe it or not, you scarcely have to clean at all. You can get by, just dusting once in a while. Your biggest responsibility may be to get your food delivered to you. People who live alone, and are ill, sometimes get into the dangerous habit of skipping meals. Don't let yourself do this! If you need help with preparing food, call family, friends, or your local Meals on Wheels.

Be flexible. After you have made a rigid list of both essential and important housework, and been creative in your search for short cuts, it is time to let yourself be a bit more flexible. You probably have some silly little jobs that mean a lot to you, like Vera's self-imposed Christmas card list. If completing such jobs makes you happy, don't skip the essential jobs, but skip some of the important ones. Doing what you choose to do will raise your spirits.

Before she was able to work again in her outdoor garden, Nikki's husband built her an indoor greenhouse. It was a lovely, life-affirming gift for a woman who cares deeply for flowers.

Perhaps for you a clean bedroom is an anti-depressant. If so, put your bedroom on the top of your priority list. Pay for a cleaning person, ask a friend to help, or let it be the first job you do whenever you feel well enough.

If sewing or gardening is relaxing for you, fine. Otherwise, skip those jobs. They are not essential. Decide your own priorities and then look for the short-cuts.

Take your time. You can no longer clean an entire house or apartment in one day. Do what you can do easily, and then be happy with what you have done rather than bitter or guilty that you couldn't do more.

When you have extra energy and are not hurting, don't waste the whole day on housework. Healthy days should bring enjoyment as well as accomplishment.

Get help. When you can't do all the work you used to do, you need help from partners, children, other relatives, friends, and hired employees. If you can afford household help, hire a person to do your housework or get a cleaning service. Hired help is almost always preferable, because they will do what you ask. You are still in charge.

Unless you are a superlative housecleaner who has always refused to be satisfied with the labor of others, you will find that most people hired to do housecleaning are quicker and more thorough than you imagined possible. And they don't tell you what to do!

You need help from your partner and your children, even when you have paid house cleaners. Remember Louise's sad story: "I hurt in every joint in my body and was so tired ... I hid my pain from the family, and when it was too bad I'd lock myself in the bedroom and cry." Denying that she was not Wonder Woman, she continued to do the housework, her job, and volunteer activities. Her family never understood, even when she was close to death, how much she needed their help. Perhaps, no matter what she did, her husband would have left and her children would have remained demanding, but she didn't give them a chance to be supportive and helpful.

The first rule with family members is: Don't hide your pain and incapacitation, and do have expectations that your family will come through for you! Bring your spouse, your mother or father, an older child, or a friend to a meeting of your lupus support group. They will learn from others that you are not the only patient who requires help.

When you have settled on a physician you like and trust, introduce your family to her. Get books on lupus from your nearest health bookstore. Health bookstores are important assets for everyone. You'll find information in these stores that simply isn't available in the average bookstore or library. Most of the stores do a large mail-order business, which is very helpful if there is no such store in your area.

Your family may love you dearly, but they may not like housework. Even in today's egalitarian society, a lot of men do little in the house, while thinking they do a lot. They may battle or procrastinate when asked to do more. It is not entirely their fault. As boys, they were not taught to be caretakers. Even if they helped their mothers, their idea of "being a man" was to sit in front of the TV, as their fathers did, until dinner was served, and then leave while the women did the dishes. Women, when they were little girls, helped their mothers, and learned from their mothers that they would grow up to be responsible for

taking care of a home and family. They played house and practiced care-taking skills with their dolls. If you are lucky, your
partner is a modern man who knows how to cook, clean, and
care for children.

If you are not getting the help you need, re-read Chapter 27
and practice assertiveness. Then don't get out of bed until the
family has the housework under control! Especially important, don't get out of bed to be the Big Boss of the jobs. Praise
whatever they do, knowing that their self-esteem and compas-
sion will increase as they unite to help you.

If you are very sick, your partner may be forced to take
complete charge of your home. Don't sabotage his authority
by giving unsolicited advice and criticism. Unless your body
is involved, as in receiving a massage, let him do things his
way. That may be hard for you, if you have always been the
homemaker, but remember that you will become healthier in
the future. Your partner will willingly relinquish the job of
head cook and bottle-washer, when you are well enough to take
it back.

Other helpers. Even if everyone sharing your home is
extremely helpful, you probably need a back-up support system. A husband who works full-time can't do everything.
Children will help, but they have their own agendas, especially
as they become old enough to be competent. Little ones wish
to help and are not too useful. Older ones have important lives
of their own.

If you have no family, you need all the help you can get
from friends and social services.

If your children are very young and your lupus symptoms
are severe, you may not be able to care for them safely. Pre-
school and day care are options, unless a loving relative is willing to keep the young children in her own home.

You have made a list of necessary tasks, and now you need
to add to that list the names and phone numbers of everyone

who is willing to help you. The longer the list of volunteers the better, because it is easier to keep people helping if they don't have to help too often. Phone friends and relatives, and read them the list of jobs you need done, or get a friend to phone for you. When a person offers to help, write that name beside the task. The list now may look like this:

Grocery shopping (Friday ... Jeanne),

Library (once a week ... Dean)

Computer (when it won't work ... May)

Back rubs (I'll call when I want one ... Moira)

Meals (Yvonne, Caroline, and Jo.) Can you think of anything lovelier than to have three friends offering to bring a meal?

Emotional support ... 10 friends!

Making phone calls to ask for help for yourself may be difficult. Most of us have been trained to "do it yourself," and not ask for help. That was possible when you were physically independent. During any phase of your disease when you cannot do for yourself, put your scruples aside.

On your lists of needs and wants, be sure to add emotional support. Good friends are assets to be treasured. Pick one or two, not in your family, who know how to listen, care about you, and are honest with you. Families are fine, too, but they tend to get involved in your troubles, or smother you with their attempts to solve your problems. You also need friends who laugh with you. If you live alone, friends are especially important.

Invite friends to visit you. As Gregory said, "When I got around to telling my friends what had been happening to me, they rallied for me. That was the only bright spot ... I found out how many good friends I have! People dropped by to take me out for a bowl of soup or just to talk."

As you find people who are willing to help you, be honest about your likes and dislikes, which may change from day to day. As Tamara said, "Sometimes a massage is wonderful and at other times it causes even more pain." The same is true of loud music, long conversations, card games, or almost any activity. Explain that lupus symptoms come and go, so you can't predict when you need help most. Make a list of people who are willing to be phoned at a moment's notice, if you suddenly need help.

Relatives and friends, even those who are younger than you, sometimes make the mistake of acting as if they are your parents, and you are a somewhat retarded child. The worst offenders usually are your mother (sometimes your father), your brothers and sisters, and your own children. They tell you what to do, and they try to think for you. "What you really need is to go back to work and get your mind off your problems." "You are too hot in this room. I'll open a window." "I think you should stop steroids and use more vitamins." "I have a friend who has a friend who says that licorice root will cure you." "You must have more exercise."

There is nothing like a chronic illness to bring out the advice-givers of the world. The old and the sick have had to put up with such annoying pseudo-parenting for years. The hardest thing for some helpers to learn is that sick people, unless their minds no longer work, are able to be in charge of their own lives.

When someone overwhelms you with unwanted advice, this may be her way of saying, "I am worried about you." A kind response is, "You are worried about me, aren't you? I'm worried about myself, too." It is always safe to say, "Thank you," to their advice, and change the subject. Sometimes you may add with a smile, "Hey, my kidneys are lousy but my thinker is still healthy." Or, "Thanks for the advice. My partner and I will consider it."

If a helper is a nuisance, set limits. "I appreciate your help, and I'll phone you when I need something, or feel like having company." You can be explicit. "I don't want to discuss with you either religion or politics, because we don't agree on these subjects." Or, "When you visit me, please don't bring me your complaints about our family."

If a visitor is wearying or toxic, and will not change, don't spend time with her. You have a right to protect yourself from such people.

Don't underestimate the help you need. Your symptoms are real, your disease is a bad one, and you may need help for quite a while. On the other hand, don't overestimate the help you need. In the long run you will be healthier and happier if you do as much as you can. For your own sake, you don't want to allow your chronic disease to become chronic idleness.

When you have set your priorities, eliminated the frill jobs, found short cuts, and enlisted the help you need, what might your days be like?

Mornings. If you wake up stiff, sore, and lethargic, don't stay in bed. Take a warm bath or shower and a short, easy walk or do tai chi or some other non-strenuous exercises. Just moving around can loosen up your body.

Give yourself a leisurely hour of breakfast, with radio, television, or the morning newspaper. Many people were taught in childhood that resting is self-indulgent, and that work must come before play. Such people find resting to be "uncomfortable" or somehow wrong, even when they are sick. You may have to teach yourself to enjoy relaxing and doing nothing. However, if you are happier doing a bit of housework as soon as you are up, go ahead.

If you are employed outside your home, you may want to wake up earlier than necessary, so that you can be leisurely rather than rushed, as you drink your coffee and get dressed.

If you awaken depressed, don't plan that you will be depressed all day; and don't stay in bed. As Maria said, "That nurse at Stanford, long ago, taught me that no matter how you feel, you should get dressed and put on make-up every day."

There is a good reason for this. Behaving as if you are well, including doing the activities you did when well, actually makes you feel better.

If you are not depressed, it can be lovely to stay in bed once in a while, with a radio and a good book, especially after the children have left for school.

Noontimes are for indoor activities, away from the sun. If you don't want to be cooped up at home, drive to a mall and walk where the sun can't reach you.

One way to keep in touch with friends is to invite them to share lunch with you, at the mall or at your home. Ask visitors to bring their own sandwiches or salads, if you are not up to making them.

Afternoons are good times for activities and social contact. If you belong to a bridge club, find a substitute who is willing to play when you are unable to be there. That way you still belong to the group. If you used to golf or play tennis with a group of friends, continue to meet them for lunch even though you can't play. Keep involved in every group that is meaningful to you.

Join an afternoon group: quilt makers, discussion groups, or whatever would interest you. Volunteer for community services, as Vera does. Your local newspaper and the Chamber of Commerce have lists of charitable organizations in your community. When you join a group, explain that you may have to miss meetings when you don't feel well enough to attend.

When you ache, are exhausted, or just don't feel well enough to do anything, get a massage, facial, or have your hair and nails done. Pamper yourself.

Twilight and **Evenings** may be your best time of day. If you love the beach by day, you'll love it at twilight. You can be in your garden or at a local park, as soon as the sun starts to set.

Take a nap before dinner or after you come home from work. A nap will give you a second wind for the evening hours.

Find a way to make quality time with your partner and your children or, if you are feeling too sick to enjoy them, plop them in front of the TV while you give yourself "alone time."

If your joints are hurting, take a hot bath before bed. Don't exercise at night, because exercise can keep you from falling asleep. If your bed makes your joints ache, because the mattress is too hard, get an "egg crate" mattress cover and use lots of pillows. Pain medicine taken at bedtime helps you get through the night without disruption from your pain.

Morning, noon, or evening, what special activities enrich your life? Here are some reported by the men and women who told their stories:

Gregory: I'm not interested in housework, so I keep everything simple. What's important to me is bicycling and sailing!

Maria: I was an outdoor person who enjoyed the sun and swimming, but now I have indoor hobbies ... ceramics and reading.

Meg: I keep busy. I work with the Senior Action Network ... picket in my wheelchair with other disabled people for better transportation for the handicapped ... listen to talking books. I got myself a scholarship to take college courses for senior citizens. Even though I can't see much, I still love to go to museums. I am given free concert tickets, and then I bribe an acquaintance to drive me to the concerts in exchange for a free ticket.

Rialta: I go out dancing and partying, even though I may be sick the next day. I am too young to spend the rest of my life doing nothing.

Pamela: I drive to the city to visit friends and relatives, and I also work part-time.

Nikki: My garden was ruined, because I didn't have energy to take care of it. I am fixing it up again, little by little. Every day just before the sun goes down, you'll find me outside, working on my garden ... and I play with my birds and chinchillas.

Joyce: I visit my mother and an ex-neighbor, who are in nursing homes. I take care of my dogs and cats. I go to garage sales and second-hand stores to find interesting odds and ends, which I use to make memory boxes and picture frames. I refinish furniture, do old-fashioned wood burning, and sew.

Dolores: When I get out of this nursing home, my boy friend and I will go gambling. Mostly, I watch TV ...and play bingo.

Vera: I belong to an organization that raises money for disabled children. I'm active in the lupus foundation and go to public lectures on lupus.

Tom: I live alone with my dog and my books. I've joined a chess club.

Beth: My time is very full, enjoying my children and pets, and gardening.

Louise: Yoga is wonderful! I have two yoga classes a week, and after the class I have lunch with some of the other participants.

Every life story in this book is unique. Some of the patients have endured terrible physical trauma and incapacitation. As Louise said, "I think I deserve to feel proud of myself, just because I still exist." The same is true of Dolores, who cared for her quadraplegic son and now lives in a nursing home, where she does not get good treatment. In spite of her disease, she found a young man who loves her and visits her daily. All of the men and women in this book are courageous. They are also lively, energetic, and creative. They have done well in building good lives in spite of lupus.

Using their lists of activities as a start, make a list of the activities that enrich your life. Write down all the things you enjoy doing, plus the activities you might like but haven't tried. Tom had no idea he'd like chess, until he read a book about it. When you have finished your list, tape it beside your bathroom mirror or next to the refrigerator, as a daily reminder to plan a happy, full day. Add new activities as you discover them. You have a right to happiness and you are the only person who can give it to you.

Happiness comes from inside. Love yourself and be good to yourself. That is the most important message in this book, and that's why it has been repeated over and over again.

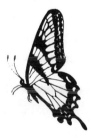

Appendix 1

The Lupus Foundation Of America
1300 Piccard Drive, Suite 200
Rockville, MD 20850-4303
301-670-9292 or 1-800-558-0121

The Lupus Foundation of America (LFA) was incorporated as a non-profit health agency in 1977. It's purpose is to assist local chapters in their efforts to provide supportive services to individuals living with lupus, to educate the public about lupus, and to support research into the causes and cure of lupus. In just twenty years, this Foundation has grown to include well over 500 constituent chapters, subchapters, and support groups, who have their own programs, services, and newsletters.

For example, the Bay Area (Northern California) chapter offers the following services, according to Jo Dewhirst, director:
Quarterly 16-page newsletter
Library, including medical articles and audio-visual material
Translations of many articles into Spanish, Chinese and Vietnamese
Semi-annual conferences
New You (Self-Image) workshops
Educational programs in English and Spanish
Medical referral list
Continuing education program for nurses and physicians
Training programs for instructors and support group representatives
Health fair
Speaker's bureau
Toll-free statewide telephone: 1-800-523-3363

To find the chapter nearest you, phone the Lupus Foundation of America. Your local chapter will introduce you to support groups in your area.

Appendix 2

Use The Internet For Information And Friendships
by Joen Fagan, Ph.D.

L et's say that you live with your lupus in a very small town in Wyoming. Reading about lupus support groups in this book makes you wish you belonged to one. You would love to have people to talk to who know what it is like to have your symptoms and problems, who have helpful suggestions, and who sympathize with what you are going through. And you could certainly use information about the latest ideas and treatments.

Suddenly, in response to your wishes, a genie appears and shows you pages from the phone book, letters from friends, and interesting articles. The genie provides you with many helpers, friends, and good information to reduce your anxiety and uncertainties, and possibly decrease your calls and visits to your doctor.

The genie really does exist. Her name is Internet or World Wide Web. Her nicknames are The Net or The Web. First, you have to acquire such a genie. Then you'll need to learn how to ask her the right questions. The genie will have so much to tell you that you may want to get a file folder right now, and mark it lupus-net.

(This is written for those who don't like or understand computers, are frightened by them, and are certain that getting on the Net may be harder than getting on the moon. If you are not a beginner, just skip to the section on Web sites.)

Start With A Free Sample. Given the many limitations on your time, money, and energy, the best place to start is with a free sample, to find out if the Net is something you want.

Find a relative or friend who is on Internet and is willing to help you. If your library has computers that go on-line, ask your librarian to show you how to use them. Or hire a high school or grammar school student to show you her setup and what she can do with it.

Get Your Own Computer. Using someone else's computer has many limitations. You can't get e-mail, be in chat groups, or use it whenever you like. If you decide you like computers, buy your own. It is a good investment for you and anyone else in your home, especially children.

If you decide to acquire your own computer, be careful not to put your choice of equipment in the hands of a computer nerd who, knowing a lot about technology but not much about you, will want you to get the very best and latest computer with dozens of gizmos that are expensive and unnecessary. For your purposes you need a computer with 8 or 16 Megabytes of RAM, a 100 Megabyte hard drive, monitor, modem, printer, and at least a six-month guarantee. A good source for a used computer is someone who wants to buy a new computer, and will throw in free lessons with the old one. Take a knowledgeable person to shop with you. A good question to ask any seller is, "What are the main problems and frustrations with this machine?"

When you've made your selection, you'll need someone to deliver the machine to your house, set it up, get it started, and teach you:

how to use the mouse, scroll, and cursor;

how to open the word processor;

how to type, print, and save files;

what to do when the computer freezes.

Select some good basic books about your computer and operating system, and study them.

Once you own a computer, you need to subscribe to an Internet Service Provider, such as America Online, Mindspring, or Netscape. At present the cost is $20 a month plus $25 start-up fee. The Provider will give you software that dials the modem-phone for you, and permits you to get e-mail and browse the Net. Pick a Provider that is known to give good service, and has a toll-free number so you don't have to pay long-distance rates. A good provider lets you ask lots of dumb questions, answers patiently, and doesn't keep you on hold for long periods of time. Don't sign a long-term contract with a Provider, because you may want to switch.

There are many little steps in the process of using a computer, and you can get stopped cold at any point if you don't know the next step, or if you put one little letter in slightly the wrong place. Learning to use a computer takes time and energy and, at times, much frustration-tolerance. You have to rely on someone who knows how to get on the Net, likes you, has patience, and is easily reachable by phone. If you plan to be taught step by step, by telephone, you need to install a separate telephone line, because you and your computer can't both be "on" at the same time.

Use The Net. If the helper is very Net-savvy, she will zoom through the instructions below and make the process of getting on the Net look easy. You won't learn that way, so sit in front of your own machine and tell her that you will do it yourself, as she tells you what to do. Practice several times, and then write down the instructions.

When working alone, expect to try a number of things from books and the instruction manual. Some will work and some will not. Half of the problem is that there are different kinds of computers, Providers, and Net browsers and search engines, and each one of them does its job a little differently. The other half of the problem is that using the Net is a skill like any other. It takes practice and the accumulation of knowledge in small doses.

Begin with something easy. After you log onto the Internet, and the main screen comes on, go to your Home or Home Page, and there you should find a box that says Net Search. If you click on it, you will find a variety of "search engines" or collections of information: Lycos, Web Crawler, Infoseek, etc. Click on any one of these sources of information to open it. It will give you a number of topics, including Health. Click on Health, and you will see a little square in which you type "lupus." Then click Search.

Yahoo is a search engine that make it especially easy to find out about lupus. It may be on the main screen of your Provider, a little box with a bright blue half-circle, and a yellow symbol that looks like a penguin or an Eskimo. Or it may be with other search engines that you get to by clicking on Net Search. Either way, when you see Yahoo, click on the symbol, wait until your screen fills, then scroll down to Health. Beside Health is Diseases and Conditions. Click on that, and wait until the list appears. Click on lupus. You will see a list of topics. Click on any of them that interests you.

WOW! You're on you way to using the Net! There are four kinds of help and information at the sites you will visit. 1. Information and articles that you can print and follow up on. 2. Chat groups, of people, all on their own computors, who converse. This resembles a conference call on the telephone. 3. Discussion groups, which are like question and answer sessions. 4. News groups or mailing lists for sending out information.

Before you get started, here are some important pieces of information:

Some of the words on the screen listing are colored differently. Some have a button beside them. Try leaving the cursor over either for a few seconds and see if you go somewhere else. Or the cursor may change color or become a little hand. Click there and you will go to another page or site.

If the new material doesn't interest you, find the little box in the upper left corner of the screen that says BACK, click on it, and you go back to where you were before.

Also note that after you have clicked on a topic, the color changes, letting you know you've already looked at that page.

If you want to come back later to a site, all you have to do is look at the top of the screen near the middle, where you'll find Bookmarks, Favorite Places, or Hot List, click on it, then click on ADD, and it will save that place. Next time you get on the Net, you can put the cursor on Bookmarks, Favorite Places, or Hot List and pull down the name of the page, and the genie will get you there immediately.

Information and articles. The easiest way to get to the Net is to find the box near the top of the Home screen that says OPEN, and click on it. Then type in one of the addresses below and hit the RETURN or ENTER key. Assuming that your Provider provides Netscape Navigator, look one fourth of the way down from the top of the page to a long, white box that says GO TO. In the box it says **http://www.(something??)** Put your cursor at the end after **(something??)**, click, and backspace to **http://www.** Now type so it reads: **http://www.yahoo.com** You must type addresses **exactly** as written, with the same capitals and small letters. Hit RETURN or ENTER. This is another way to get to Yahoo. Find Health and then Diseases, then lupus.

Another very useful search engine is WebCrawler. Go to Net Search and click on WebCrawler or OPEN and type in **http://webcrawler.com** and hit ENTER or RETURN. When it opens, don't click on Health, but put your cursor on Search and type in lupus and hit RETURN or ENTER. It will tell you there are over a thousand entries on lupus, and will start you off with twenty-five. A good place to start is to look down the list and find Nikki's Lupus Links and click on it. This will link you to just about everything worth going to.

Other good Web sites:

http://www.lupus.org/lupus is a website of the Lupus Foundation of America. Here you can find a list of chapters or a summary of current research, look at health forums, and more.

http://www.yahoo.com/health/alternative medicine is full of information.

http://www.altmedicine.com This site can get you into Medline, which carries abstracts and articles from medical journals. Check the Health News Bulletins and What's New. Then scroll down to Diet and Nutrition, Alternative Medical Systems, or whatever you like. Other good sites:

http://www.hamline.edu.lupus

http://www.lupuseanada.org

http://galaxy.einet.net/galaxy/medicine.html This is a site with extensive medical information. Under diseases and disorders, look for immunologic, which includes lupus.

http://www.rxlist.com gives you drug information, such as is found in the Physicians Desk Reference.

USENETsci.med.pharmacy is another drug information site.

It is easy to connect with chat lines on the following three sites:

http://www.mtio.com/melfa

http://www.mtio/melfa/ifacha.html

http://www.lupus.org/lupus

If you have AOL, look on the main menu for People Connection and click. There will be a big list of interests. You're not limited to lupus; look under Health and Mental Health and you'll find groups for depression, parents of children with attention-deficit disorders, etc.

When you begin talking with others on the Net, they will tell you the names of other sites. Remember, the Net is constantly changing, so what is here today may be gone tomorrow and something much better will have replaced it.

Chat groups usually have specific times to get together, but there may be someone there to talk at any time. The chat group window will show you the number of people chatting. Type in a greeting, for example, "This is my first time on the chat line," then hit Return or Enter.

At first the messages may seem confusing, because several people may be "talking" at the same time. You'll get the hang of it soon. The chat group often involves personal material, emotional reactions, and closeness.

However, be very careful about using your real name and address, and never give anyone your credit card numbers or your Provider password. You don't know who may be listening in, or whether the person wants the information for a scam. A good way to find friends is to write e-mail letters to people whose messages you especially like.

Discussion groups. These are also called forum or bulletin boards or message boards. They are like question and answer sessions. You can write out a question, and other people will answer you. You can also answer questions that others ask. Here are some good discussion sites:

http://www.yahoo.com/Health/AlternativeMedicine
http://www.mtio.com/wwwboard/wwwboard.html
http://www.lupus.org/lupus/forum/forum.html
http://www.hamline.edu/lupus/indes.htmll
news:alt.support.lupus

Next, test out news groups or mailing lists. They are like Discussion Groups, except that their letters and articles show up on your e-mail. If you sign on, you will get a lot of advertising with the information, and perhaps more e-mail than you want.

The Net is good for many things besides lupus. Look at paintings in the Louvre **http://mistral.culture.fr/louvre**
See pictures of the earth, taken from space by astronauts **http://earth.jse.nasa.gov** Visiting the net is like going to a big, strange city where there are wonderful things to see and do.

Get On E-mail. E-mail is a cross between a telephone and regular mail, and cheaper than either. You can leave messages any time at all, make long distance calls free, and you don't need to buy stamps or find a post office. A disadvantage is that not everyone has e-mail yet, but within a few years they will.

Since different Providers access e-mail differently, you will need to ask your helper to show you the steps. Ask her to show you how to: send, return, and forward letters; put letters in SAVE; make folders and put letters in them; discard letters; empty trash; use address book, including adding, changing, and deleting addresses; print letters; attach files to letters. If your Provider charges for time on, you'll want to learn to read and write e-mail off-line.

If this sounds like a lot to learn, remember that you are learning something that can give you hours of pleasure, as well as high quality support, friendship, and information. The genie really exists.

Authors

CLAUDIA PAGANO, RN, BSN, is a critical care nurse at Salinas Valley Memorial Hospital, Salinas, California. She was diagnosed with systemic lupus erythematosus in 1991 and immediately organized a lupus support group for Monterey and surrounding counties. Under her leadership, the group joined the Bay Area Lupus Foundation, which is a chapter of the Lupus Foundation of America. She has been interviewed in local newspapers and magazines, and receives referrals from physicians and other health care providers who have lupus patients requesting information and support.

MARY MCCLURE GOULDING, MSW, and her late husband, Robert L. Goulding, MD, developed Redecision psychotherapy, which they taught at their Western Institute and in many countries throughout the world. Goulding is one of three women to be honored as a major presenter at all Evolution of Psychotherapy Conferences, 1985, 1990, 1995, and in Germany in 1994. She has published 6 books.

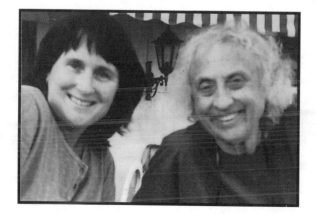

INDEX

To order books written by Pagano or Goulding

Make checks payable to:
Abiding Health Publications
P.O. Box 3828
Salinas, CA 93912

A TIME TO SAY GOOD-BYE   USA $14.00
...Moving beyond loss, 1996
by Mary McClure Goulding

CHANGING LIVES THROUGH
REDECISION THERAPY   USA $13.00
...A definitive text of psychotherapy
by Mary McClure Goulding and
Robert L. Goulding, M.D.
Revised and Updated by Mary Goulding, 1997

SWEET LOVE REMEMBERED   USA $14.00
...A life story of Bob Goulding
by Mary Goulding, 1992

LUPUS — WHAT'S IT ALL ABOUT?   USA $14.95
by Claudia Pagano and
Mary McClure Goulding, 1998

Postage and handling, one book $3.00
Two – nine books, per book $2.00
Ten or more books   postage free

California residents add sales tax: 7.25%